CLINICAL TRIALS
AUDIT PREPARATION

CLINICAL TRIALS AUDIT PREPARATION
A Guide for Good Clinical Practice (GCP) Inspections

VERA MIHAJLOVIC-MADZAREVIC

Global Research Pharma Canada, Inc.
Thornhill, Ontario, Canada

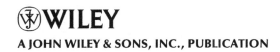

A JOHN WILEY & SONS, INC., PUBLICATION

Published by John Wiley & Sons, Inc., Hoboken, New Jersey.
Published simultaneously in Canada.

For general information on our other products and services or for technical support, please contact our Customer Care Department within the United States at (800) 762-2974, outside the United States at (317) 572-3993 or fax (317) 572-4002.

Wiley also publishes its books in a variety of electronic formats. Some content that appears in print may not be available in electronic formats. For more information about Wiley products, visit our web site at www.wiley.com.

Library of Congress Cataloging-in-Publication Data:

Mihajlovic-Madzarevic, Vera.
    Clinical trials audit preparation : a guide for good clinical practice (GCP) inspections / Vera Mihajlovic-Madzarevic.
        p.   ;   cm.
    Includes index.
    ISBN 978-0-470-24885-0 (cloth)
    1. Drugs–Testing–Auditing.   2. Medical audit.   I. Title.
    [DNLM: 1. Clinical Trials as Topic–standards.   2. Guideline Adherence–standards.
   3. Management Audit.   4. Quality Control.   QV 771 M636c 2010]
    RM301.27.M54   2010
    615.5′80724–dc22
                                        2009027971

10 9 8 7 6 5 4 3 2 1

PREFACE

GCP inspections of clinical trial sites are the challenges that clinical research faces in demonstrating data credibility and patient safety. However, I found in my clinical research experience that audits are a tedious but nevertheless necessary activity to assure that all parties do their job right.

Being a clinical scientist and third party auditor allowed me to understand the struggles in clinical research (CR) and quality assurance (QA). Although CR and QA are independent activities (we do not talk to each other unless necessary) they have interdependent tasks. The auditor should know the challenges of the clinical research associate/monitor, and vice versa. Understanding the objectives of each other's tasks will allow the clinical work to proceed smoothly.

In the last 15 years since ICH GCP was issued as an International Guidance for clinical research, the pharmaceutical research-based industry as well as academic research institutions had to realign all their activities to remain "compliant" to regulations. The setting of clear and uniform standards raised the bar for clinical research and development (R&D); however, it also increased the cost to staggering levels.

During my preregulatory inspections of clinical trial sites and sponsors as well as GLP labs, a constant issue was always present—the dread of the inspected facility of the possible findings and their consequences.

Many times while performing inspections I was asked "Are we in compliance?" or "Do you see something serious?" My logical thought was "Will I be able to find all possible sources of noncompliance before the FDA inspector comes?" Could I provide assurance to my client that everything was OK?

Obviously, some of my clients are happy to see me and eager to walk though the inspection, learning and uncovering all possible issues. However, others dislike my presence, thinking that I will point a finger at people who did things wrong and who thus may lose their jobs. At that point I feel isolated and unwanted, but badly needed.

The best part is at the end of the inspection, when we all sit down to dissect the results and the clinical teams start to understand the meaning of the findings and accept suggestions to achieve compliance. Finally, we all shake hands and, with a smile, we go home after long days of document hunting and endless reading.

The writing of the report is another story. When I write my inspection report, it does not look like a Form 483; it is a "catharsis" for my client. I summarize hundreds of findings in a tabulated manner where the last column is "Suggested Remedial Action." I point out the noncompliance and how to get back on track. That is a relief to my clients, since action can be taken immediately to ensure future compliance.

Of course, it would be childish to suggest that all noncompliance can be remediated: some noncompliance issues are based on the complete misunderstanding of the requirement or regulation, and on strong opinions based on old school medicine.

With this book I was given the task of putting together the world of the regulator, the sponsor of clinical research, and the investigators. As a professional development instructor and former university teacher, I understand that we cannot start speaking of a particular topic without first seeing the big picture, and where that topic fits in and the implications and future consequences of the issue discussed. I do not take anything for granted until it is explained and understood. Therefore, it was very important that with the first chapters I review compliance to what, and then compliance by whom, and finally how to achieve compliance. Understanding the drug development process is also a must, since the reader needs to be on the same page to understand the inspection process. The processes described in this book are part of the FDA BIMO compliance programs 7348.810 and 7348.811 that are publicly available.

The challenge in writing this book was to present the subjects objectively to avoid the boredom inherent in a dry topic as GCP compliance. Therefore, I covered the responsibilities of the parties in clinical research according to GCP and 21 CFR 312, and other applicable requirements and utilized examples as much as possible. The biggest challenge was that every time I thought I had finished, new things happened in the clinical research world that I had to include, and every review was an update until I said this is it, for now. I am already thinking of the next edition and how things will change in the coming years.

We have to move forward in clinical research and in how therapeutic products are developed. Ten to twelve years for development and billions of dollars is too much for a failure rate of more than 75%, and changes are coming soon. Read the FDAAA (http://www.fda.gov/oc/initiatives/advance/fdaaa/accomplishments.html) for current insight.

Having the privilege to work in basic scientific research, medicine, clinical research and development and being a scientist, I was able to present clearly issues from product discovery to market and write about them from the compliance point of view.

Another topic that I consider extremely informative is the analysis of warning letters. As we go through the regulatory findings we can easily see where the failures in compliance are and what may be missing. I do suggest that all clinical research professionals read the FDA warning letters to clinical investigators, sponsors, and institutional review boards as they appear in the FDA website, since they point out issues that arose after detailed review of data and documents; this will increase the reader's pool of regulatory knowledge.

Lastly, I formulated several key questions in understanding GCP compliance to clarify topics that may pop up when reading the guidance.

The footnote references are a pivotal part of this book; the reader has been provided some of the documents referred to in the footnotes in the appendixes.

My last bit of advice is that before implementing processes or procedures (SOPs), read the code of federal regulations applicable to your activity or product. Also, go to the source, and never rely on interpretations or guidance that may be only the opinion of one party. See the whole picture, and then you will understand why.

VERA MIHAJLOVIC-MADZAREVIC

Thornhill, Ontario, Canada
January 2010

INTRODUCTION

Clinical trials are conducted in humans to determine safety, tolerability, and efficacy of potential therapeutic products. Those trials have to be conducted in compliance with specific regulatory requirements and Good Clinical Practice to demonstrate that patient's rights, safety, and well-being, as well as data credibility are ensured.

Internal sponsor audits together with FDA regulatory inspections of clinical trial activities are essential to assure compliance with SOPs, GCPs, and established regulatory requirements.

This book intends to summarize specific aspects of drug development as well as present in a clear and concise manner the principles of drug development and Good Clinical Practices.

It is very important that the clinical research stakeholder (sponsor, investigator, or member of an Institutional Review Board) understands the basic principles of the GCP guideline, since it highlights the spirit of the requirements for clinical trials. The FDA, although it did not implement ICH/GCP into its regulations, is fully observant.

Following the principles of GCP will allow stakeholders to focus their activities in a compliant fashion. Understanding the regulatory requirements established in the FDA code of federal regulations, particularly 21 CFR 11, 50, 54, 56, 312, 314, 320, 601, 812, and 814, will allow the research professional to establish proper processes and procedures to ensure compliance for FDA regulated trials.

This book will guide the reader through the extensive foundation of knowledge that is necessary to understand and be prepared for the task of conducting clinical investigations in human subjects.

Since its implementation, the FDA Bioresearch Monitoring Program has been in charge of GCP inspections of clinical trial investigative sites, sponsors, Institutional Review Boards, and Contract Research Organizations. The processes and procedures that the inspector follows are publicly available in the *FDA Compliance Program Guidance Manual*. However, this book assists readers to understand how the process works, who is inspected and why, and what are the consequences of an inspection. An in-depth analysis of warning letters gives the reader an insight of what is essentially going wrong, and where stakeholders have to improve.

BACKGROUND HISTORY ON CLINICAL RESEARCH STANDARDS

Clinical research and development has undergone extensive changes in the last decades, adapting to a continuously changing regulatory framework. With the need to expand the applicability of clinical trial data gathered internationally, it was recognized that common grounds should be established for global research and development of therapeutic products.

Large R&D-oriented pharmaceutical companies initially implemented their own R&D standards and internal processes aimed at local regulatory requirements for submission purposes. In the last few decades, before new guidelines were set into place, clinical trials were mostly conducted at a local level, and the industry had to spend additional resources and time to satisfy every country-specific requirement. There was no unified standard for the conduct of clinical trials; therefore, standards were set up independently by regulatory bodies to be consistent with the Declaration of Helsinki.[1]

The Declaration of Helsinki was adopted by the 18th World Medical Association Assembly in 1964 and outlined the basis for the ethical principles for medical research involving human subjects, serving as the main document for the conduct of medical research. The fundamentals of the declaration were set in the Nuremberg Code[2] after the Nuremberg tribunal exposed medical research crimes committed during the Second World War.

In the United States, on April 18, 1979, the National Commission for the Protection of Human Subjects of Biomedical and Behavioral Research issued the Belmont Report,[3] which identified the basic ethical principles that underlined the conduct of biomedical and behavioral research involving human subjects and developed guidelines that should be followed to assure that such research is conducted in accordance with those principles.

Both documents focused on subjects' rights and safety as the main concern; however, they were inadequate on setting a standard for data quality, accuracy, and integrity.

It is reasonable to understand that data quality was not the objective of those documents since they are mostly an extension of the Nuremberg Code, which focused purposely on subjects' rights and safety.

Therefore, after observing a great procedural and implemental disparity in clinical research, the need was identified for a process that will be internationally accepted to set the guidelines for the conduct of human research, taking into account both aspects of clinical research: subject's rights and safety, and data quality, accuracy, and validity.

The International Conference on Harmonisation of Technical Requirements for Registration of Pharmaceuticals for Human Use issued the *ICH Harmonised Tripartite Guideline for Good Clinical Practice E6(R1)*[4] on June 10, 1996. In this document the industry and stakeholders, for the first time, have an international ethical and scientific quality standard for designing, conducting, recording, and reporting trials that involve the participation of human subjects. This document addresses both aspects of clinical research: patients' rights and safety and data quality, accuracy, and integrity.

---

[1] World Medical Association Declaration of Helsinki: Ethical Principles for Medical Research Involving Human Subjects. See Appendix C at the end of this book.

[2] See Appendix D at the end of this book for a copy of the Nuremberg Code.

[3] See Appendix E for a copy of this report.

[4] International Conference on Harmonisation of Technical Requirements for Registration of Pharmaceuticals for Human Use. *ICH Harmonised Tripartite Guideline for Good Clinical Practice E6(R1)*, June 10, 1996.

GLOSSARY

The glossary in this book is aligned with the definitions provided in the ICH/GCP document.[5]

Adverse Drug Reaction (ADR): In the preapproval clinical experience with a new medicinal product or its new usages, particularly as the therapeutic dose(s) may not be established: all noxious and unintended responses to a medicinal product related to any dose should be considered adverse drug reactions. The phrase responses to a medicinal product means that a causal relationship between a medicinal product and an adverse event is at least a reasonable possibility; that is, the relationship cannot be ruled out.

Regarding marketed medicinal products: a response to a drug which is noxious and unintended and which occurs at doses normally used in humans for prophylaxis, diagnosis, or therapy of diseases or for modification of physiological function (see the *ICH Guideline for Clinical Safety Data Management: Definitions and Standards for Expedited Reporting*).

Adverse Event (AE): Any untoward medical occurrence in a patient or clinical investigation subject administered a pharmaceutical product and which does not necessarily have a causal relationship with this treatment. An adverse event (AE) can therefore be any unfavorable and unintended sign (including an abnormal laboratory finding), symptom, or disease temporally associated with the use of a medicinal (investigational) product, whether or not related to the medicinal (investigational) product (see the *ICH Guideline for Clinical Safety Data Management: Definitions and Standards for Expedited Reporting*).

Applicable Regulatory Requirement(s): Any law(s) and regulation(s) addressing the conduct of clinical trials of investigational products.

Approval (in relation to Institutional Review Boards): The affirmative decision of the IRB that the clinical trial has been reviewed and may be conducted at the institution site within the constraints set forth by the IRB, the institution, Good Clinical Practice (GCP), and the applicable regulatory requirements.

Audit: A systematic and independent examination of trial-related activities and documents to determine whether the evaluated trial-related activities were conducted, and the data were recorded, analyzed, and accurately reported according to the protocol, sponsor's standard operating procedures (SOPs), Good Clinical Practice (GCP), and the applicable regulatory requirement(s).

Audit Certificate: A declaration of confirmation by the auditor that an audit has taken place.

Audit Report: A written evaluation by the sponsor's auditor of the results of the audit.

Audit Trail: Documentation that allows reconstruction of the course of events.

Blinding/Masking: A procedure in which one or more parties to the trial are kept unaware of the treatment assignment(s). Single-blinding usually refers to the subject(s) being unaware,

---

[5] *Guidance for Industry—E6 Good Clinical Practice: Consolidated Guidance*, U.S. Department of Health and Human Services, Food and Drug Administration, Center for Drug Evaluation and Research (CDER) and Center for Biologics Evaluation and Research (CBER), April 1996 ICH.

and double-blinding usually refers to the subject(s), investigator(s), monitor, and, in some cases, data analyst(s) being unaware of the treatment assignment(s).

Case Report Form (CRF): A printed, optical, or electronic document designed to record all of the protocol required information to be reported to the sponsor on each trial subject.

Clinical Trial/Study: Any investigation in human subjects intended to discover or verify the clinical, pharmacological, and/or other pharmacodynamic effects of an investigational product(s), and/or to identify any adverse reactions to an investigational product(s), and/or to study absorption, distribution, metabolism, and excretion of an investigational product(s) with the object of ascertaining its safety and/or efficacy. The terms clinical trial and clinical study are synonymous.

Clinical Trial/Study Report: A written description of a trial/study of any therapeutic, prophylactic, or diagnostic agent conducted in human subjects, in which the clinical and statistical description, presentations, and analyses are fully integrated into a single report (see the *ICH Guideline for Structure and Content of Clinical Study Reports*).

Comparator (Product): An investigational or marketed product (i.e., active control), or placebo, used as a reference in a clinical trial.

Compliance (in relation to trials): Adherence to all the trial-related requirements, Good Clinical Practice (GCP) requirements, and the applicable regulatory requirements.

Confidentiality: Prevention of disclosure, to other than authorized individuals, of a sponsor's proprietary information or of a subject's identity.

Contract: A written, dated, and signed agreement between two or more involved parties that sets out any arrangements on delegation and distribution of tasks and obligations and, if appropriate, on financial matters. The protocol may serve as the basis of a contract.

Coordinating Committee: A committee that a sponsor may organize to coordinate the conduct of a multicenter trial.

Coordinating Investigator: An investigator assigned the responsibility for the coordination of investigators at different centers participating in a multicenter trial.

Contract Research Organization (CRO): A person or an organization (commercial, academic, or other) contracted by the sponsor to perform one or more of a sponsor's trial-related duties and functions.

Direct Access: Permission to examine, analyze, verify, and reproduce any records and reports that are important to evaluation of a clinical trial. Any party (e.g., domestic and foreign regulatory authorities, sponsor's monitors and auditors) with direct access should take all reasonable precautions within the constraints of the applicable regulatory requirement(s) to maintain the confidentiality of subjects' identities and sponsor's proprietary information.

Documentation: All records, in any form (including, but not limited to, written, electronic, magnetic, and optical records, and scans, X rays, and electrocardiograms) that describe or record the methods, conduct, and/or results of a trial, the factors affecting a trial, and the actions taken.

Essential Documents: Documents that individually and collectively permit evaluation of the conduct of a study and the quality of the data produced (see point 8 in *Essential Documents for the Conduct of a Clinical Trial*).

Independent Data Monitoring Committee (IDMC) (Data and Safety Monitoring Board, Monitoring Committee, Data Monitoring Committee): An independent data monitoring committee that may be established by the sponsor to assess at intervals the progress of a clinical trial, the safety data, and the critical efficacy endpoints, and to recommend to the sponsor whether to continue, modify, or stop a trial.

Impartial Witness: A person who is independent of the trial, who cannot be unfairly influenced by people involved with the trial, who attends the informed consent process if the subject or the subject's legally acceptable representative cannot read, and who reads the informed consent form and any other written information supplied to the subject.

Independent Ethics Committee (IEC): An independent body (a review board or a committee, institutional, regional, national, or supranational), constituted of medical professionals and nonmedical members, whose responsibility it is to ensure the protection of the rights, safety, and well-being of human subjects involved in a trial and to provide public assurance of that protection by, among other things, reviewing and approving/providing favorable opinion on the trial protocol, the suitability of the investigator(s), facilities, and the methods and material to be used in obtaining and documenting informed consent of the trial subjects.

The legal status, composition, function, operations and regulatory requirements pertaining to Independent Ethics Committees may differ among countries but should allow the Independent Ethics Committee to act in agreement with GCP as described in this guideline.

Informed Consent: A process by which a subject voluntarily confirms his/her willingness to participate in a particular trial, after having been informed of all aspects of the trial that are relevant to the subject's decision to participate. Informed consent is documented by means of a written, signed and dated informed consent form.

Inspection: The act by a regulatory authority(ies) of conducting an official review of documents, facilities, records, and any other resources that are deemed by the authority(ies) to be related to the clinical trial and that may be located at the site of the trial, at the sponsor's and/or contract research organization's (CRO's) facilities, or at other establishments deemed appropriate by the regulatory authority(ies).

Institution (medical): Any public or private entity or agency or medical or dental facility where clinical trials are conducted.

Institutional Review Board (IRB): An independent body constituted of medical, scientific, and nonscientific members, whose responsibility is to ensure the protection of the rights, safety, and well-being of human subjects involved in a trial by, among other things, reviewing, approving, and providing continuing review of trial protocol and amendments and of the methods and material to be used in obtaining and documenting informed consent of the trial subjects.

Interim Clinical Trial/Study Report: A report of intermediate results and their evaluation based on analyses performed during the course of a trial.

Investigational Product: A pharmaceutical form of an active ingredient or placebo being tested or used as a reference in a clinical trial, including a product with a marketing authorization when used or assembled (formulated or packaged) in a way different from the approved form, or when used for an unapproved indication, or when used to gain further information about an approved use.

Investigator: A person responsible for the conduct of the clinical trial at a trial site. If a trial is conducted by a team of individuals at a trial site, the investigator is the responsible leader of the team and may be called the principal investigator.

Investigator/Institution: An expression meaning "the investigator and/or institution, where required by the applicable regulatory requirements."

Investigator's Brochure: A compilation of the clinical and nonclinical data on the investigational product(s) which is relevant to the study of the investigational product(s) in human subjects.

Legally Acceptable Representative: An individual or juridical or other body authorized under applicable law to consent, on behalf of a prospective subject, to the subject's participation in the clinical trial.

Monitoring: The act of overseeing the progress of a clinical trial, and of ensuring that it is conducted, recorded, and reported in accordance with the protocol, standard operating procedures (SOPs), Good Clinical Practice (GCP), and the applicable regulatory requirement(s).

Monitoring Report: A written report from the monitor to the sponsor after each site visit and/or other trial-related communication according to the sponsor's SOPs.

Multicentre Trial: A clinical trial conducted according to a single protocol but at more than one site and therefore carried out by more than one investigator.

Nonclinical Study: Biomedical studies not performed on human subjects.

Opinion (in relation to Independent Ethics Committee): The judgment and/or the advice provided by an Independent Ethics Committee (IEC).

Original Medical Record: See **Source Documents**.

Protocol: A document that describes the objective(s), design, methodology, statistical considerations, and organization of a trial. The protocol usually also gives the background and rationale for the trial, but these could be provided in other protocol referenced documents. Throughout the ICH GCP guideline the term protocol refers to protocol and protocol amendments.

Protocol Amendment: A written description of a change(s) to or formal clarification of a protocol.

Quality Assurance (QA): All those planned and systematic actions that are established to ensure that the trial is performed and the data are generated, documented (recorded), and reported in compliance with Good Clinical Practice (GCP) and the applicable regulatory requirement(s).

Quality Control (QC): The operational techniques and activities undertaken within the quality assurance system to verify that the requirements for quality of the trial-related activities have been fulfilled.

Randomization: The process of assigning trial subjects to treatment or control groups using an element of chance to determine the assignments in order to reduce bias.

Regulatory Authorities: Bodies having the power to regulate. In the ICH GCP guideline the expression "regulatory authorities" includes the authorities that review submitted clinical data and those that conduct inspections. These bodies are sometimes referred to as competent authorities.

Serious Adverse Event (SAE) or Serious Adverse Drug Reaction (Serious ADR): Any untoward medical occurrence that, at any dose, results in death, is life-threatening, requires inpatient hospitalization or prolongation of existing hospitalization, results in persistent or significant disability/incapacity, or is a congenital anomaly/birth defect.

Source Data: All information in original records and certified copies of original records of clinical findings, observations, or other activities in a clinical trial necessary for the reconstruction and evaluation of the trial. Source data are contained in source documents (original records or certified copies).

Source Documents: Original documents, data, and records (e.g., hospital records, clinical and office charts, laboratory notes, memoranda, subjects' diaries or evaluation checklists, pharmacy dispensing records, recorded data from automated instruments, copies or transcriptions certified after verification as being accurate copies, microfiches, photographic negatives, microfilm or magnetic media, X rays, subject files, and records kept at the pharmacy, at the laboratories, and at medico-technical departments involved in the clinical trial).

Sponsor: An individual, company, institution, or organization that takes responsibility for the initiation, management, and/or financing of a clinical trial.

Sponsor–Investigator: An individual who both initiates and conducts, alone or with others, a clinical trial, and under whose immediate direction the investigational product is administered to, dispensed to, or used by a subject. The term does not include any person other than an individual (e.g., it does not include a corporation or an agency). The obligations of a sponsor–investigator include both those of a sponsor and those of an investigator.

Standard Operating Procedures (SOPs): Detailed, written instructions to achieve uniformity of the performance of a specific function.

Subinvestigator: Any individual member of the clinical trial team designated and supervised by the investigator at a trial site to perform critical trial-related procedures and/or to make important trial-related decisions (e.g., associates, residents, research fellows). See also **Investigator**.

Subject/Trial Subject: An individual who participates in a clinical trial, either as a recipient of the investigational product(s) or as a control.

Subject Identification Code: A unique identifier assigned by the investigator to each trial subject to protect the subject's identity and used in lieu of the subject's name when the investigator reports adverse events and/or other trial-related data.

Trial Site: The location(s) where trial-related activities are actually conducted.

Unexpected Adverse Drug Reaction: An adverse reaction, the nature or severity of which is not consistent with the applicable product information (e.g., Investigator's Brochure for an unapproved investigational product or package insert/summary of product characteristics for an approved product).

Vulnerable Subjects: Individuals whose willingness to volunteer in a clinical trial may be unduly influenced by the expectation, whether justified or not, of benefits associated with participation, or of a retaliatory response from senior members of a hierarchy in case of refusal to participate. Examples are members of a group with a hierarchical structure, such as medical, pharmacy, dental, and nursing students, subordinate hospital and laboratory personnel, employees of the pharmaceutical industry, members of the armed forces, and persons kept in detention. Other vulnerable subjects include patients with incurable diseases, persons in nursing homes, unemployed or impoverished persons, patients in emergency situations, ethnic minority groups, homeless persons, nomads, refugees, minors, and those incapable of giving consent.

Well-being (of the trial subjects): The physical and mental integrity of the subjects participating in a clinical trial.

CHAPTER 1

GOOD CLINICAL PRACTICE AND THERAPEUTIC PRODUCT DEVELOPMENT

This chapter provides the background information necessary to understand the universal basis of the inspectional strategies for clinical trials. Consequently, to be able to understand the purpose and background of an inspection, it is very important to comprehend Good Clinical Practice (GCP) and its applicability in real situations in clinical trials.

GCP will not teach or direct medical doctors on how to run a clinic, but rather will guide all parties involved in clinical research (the sponsors, the investigator, and the ethics boards) on what practices and procedures will ensure patient safety and data credibility.

It is very important that all personnel involved in clinical trials are properly trained and updated on GCP and understand the end implications of noncompliant activities in clinical research.

Together with GCP the reader should understand the FDA drug development process, where the regulator, observing GCP, outlines country-specific procedures and requirements to ensure compliance.

Also, this book discusses the applicability of GCP in postmarketing studies that have become increasingly necessary for the continuous evaluation of safety and efficacy of a marketed therapeutic product. The new approach of regulators worldwide seeking more postmarketing research took a definite turn with implementation of the FDAAA (FDA Amendment Act) in 2007, where the agency was provided with more enforcement power to direct sponsors holding a market authorization to sell a drug product, to conduct Phase IV clinical trials to further support safety and efficacy.

Initially, to ensure compliance to standards and regulatory requirements, all parties in clinical research have to implement quality assurance (QA) processes as needed. This book discusses, in a concise manner, what QA means for all clinical research parties involved and how to implement an efficient QA program to act preemptively on a regulatory inspection.

Clinical Trials Audit Preparation: A Guide for Good Clinical Practice (GCP) Inspections, by Vera Mihajlovic-Madzarevic
Copyright © 2010 John Wiley & Sons, Inc.

The main topics discussed in this chapter are:

- Good Clinical Practice in clinical research
- Clinical development of therapeutic products in the United States
- Phase IV studies and GCP
- Quality assurance in clinical research

1.1 GOOD CLINICAL PRACTICE IN CLINICAL RESEARCH

1.1.1 Definition

Good Clinical Practice is a standard for the design, conduct, performance, monitoring, auditing, recording, analyses, and reporting of clinical trials that provides assurance that the data and reported results are credible and accurate, and that the rights, integrity, and confidentiality of trial subjects are protected.

The main elements of GCP are (1) the **subject's** rights, welfare, and confidentiality and (2) **data** validity, integrity, and credibility.

1.1.2 GCP Compliance

Compliance with GCP provides public assurance that the rights, safety, and well-being of trial subjects are protected in consistency with the principles that have their origin in the Declaration of Helsinki, and that the clinical trial data are credible.

Patient safety and data credibility are the main objectives not only to GCP as a guideline, but to the FDA and other regulatory authorities as their requirements for clinical investigations on human therapeutic products.

1.1.3 GCP Objectives

The objective of GCP is stated by the document as follows:

"To provide a unified standard for the European Union (EU), Japan, and the United States to facilitate the mutual acceptance of clinical data by the regulatory authorities in these jurisdictions."

This definition applies also to all other countries that adhere to these guidelines.

These standards were adopted by most countries worldwide that have regulatory bodies that want to be integrated into the global mutual clinical data flow for submission purposes.

The FDA is <u>observant</u> of ICH/GCP guidelines (meaning that the FDA CFR precedes the guideline, but does not disagree with the principle).

It must be noted that although these guidelines should be followed by any party when generating clinical trial data that are intended to be submitted to regulatory authorities for market approval purposes, it also should be applicable to **any investigation where human subjects are participants**.

> GCP should be considered applicable to **any investigation where human subjects are participants.**

1.1.4   Principles of ICH GCP

Clinical Trial Conduct   Clinical trials should be conducted in accordance with the ethical principles that have their origin in the Declaration of Helsinki, and that are consistent with GCP and the applicable regulatory requirement(s).

Risk Assessment   Before a trial is initiated, foreseeable risks and inconveniences should be weighed against the anticipated benefit for the individual trial subject and society. A trial should be initiated and continued only if the anticipated benefits justify the risks.

Subject's Rights and Safety   The rights, safety, and well-being of the trial subjects are the most important considerations and should prevail over interests of science and society.

Background Information   All available nonclinical and clinical information on an investigational product should be adequate to support the proposed clinical trial.

Clinical Trial Protocol   Clinical trials should be scientifically sound and described in a clear, detailed protocol.

> Note that the content structure of the protocol should be consistent to a standard format to allow easy search reading and understanding.

Ethics Review and Approval   A trial should be conducted in compliance with the protocol that has received prior Institutional Review Board (IRB)/Independent Ethics Committee (IEC) approval/favorable opinion. Mainly, all documents reviewed and approved by the IRBs have to be included in the approval letter to identify precisely the study, the protocol, and other related documents.

Ethics review boards have to be duly constituted according to GCP and local requirements and should follow standard operating procedures to demonstrate adherence.

> Note that any ethics board that is not constituted and does not function according to regulatory requirements and GCP cannot issue a valid approval. From the investigator's compliance point of view (see Form 1572[1]) it is like running a clinical trial without approval.

[1]FDA Form 1572, Statement of the Investigator. Electronically available at http://www.fda.gov/downloads/AboutFDA/ReportsManualForms/Forms/UCM074728.pdf.

Medical Care of Trial Subject GCP is very clear that clinical trial personnel have to be qualified to perform the duties required. Therefore, "the medical care given to, and medical decisions made on behalf of, subjects should always be the responsibility of a qualified physician or, when appropriate, of a qualified dentist." Also if you refer to the Declaration of Helsinki this premise is consistent.

Qualifications of Clinical Trial Personnel "Each individual involved in conducting a trial should be qualified by education, training, and experience to perform his or her respective task(s)."

Informed Consent Process The informed consent process goes far beyond the consent document per se. The process itself is part of the scrutiny during an inspection. It must be demonstrated that the consent was obtained freely, without prejudice or duress: "Freely given informed consent should be obtained from every subject prior to clinical trial participation."

Data Management Once a study commences, the clinical trial data has to be collected **with extreme care and precision**. "All clinical trial information should be recorded, handled, and stored in a way that allows its accurate reporting, interpretation, and verification." The process of data management has to be described in detail in the sponsor's standard operating procedures, which also are going to be inspected.

Patient Confidentiality Patient health records are covered by strict regulations. All data that is collected for clinical trials purposes must be treated as private and confidential. "The confidentiality of records that could identify subjects should be protected, respecting the privacy and confidentiality rules in accordance with the applicable regulatory requirement(s)." The patient information and consent form should be written in accordance with local requirements and GCP to assure the participants that their identity will always be protected. Note that confidentiality of patient records and how the information is handled varies from country to country according to their laws, and the sponsor has to be very much aware of the differences.

Investigational Product Manufacturing, Handling, and Storage The sponsor is responsible for the investigational product that is being studied. "Investigational products should be manufactured, handled, and stored in accordance with applicable good manufacturing practice (GMP). They should be used in accordance with the approved protocol."

Quality Assurance Sponsors and Institutional Review Boards should implement standard procedures to ensure that the activities carried out are in compliance with GCP and regulatory requirements. As you can observe, GCP does not establish requirements for the investigator to implement SOPs. The issue of investigators and SOPs will be discussed later.

However, it is not enough to have written procedures of SOPs, since once procedures are written and implemented, **a quality assurance process** should be put in place to ensure that those activities have been carried out as per procedures and that if deviations have been observed, they are corrected and the activity well documented.

GCP requires that "systems with procedures that assure the quality of every aspect of the trial should be implemented." Investigators should follow the procedures that are described in the protocol for a clinical investigation.

However, due to the inspectional findings where investigators fail to comply with their own responsibilities as investigators (described in brief in the signed Form 1572), written standard operating procedures are being sought. This issue is also going to be discussed further since written SOPs may not assure that the investigator will not repeat noncompliant activities. Therefore, a robust QA program has to be implemented when procedures are written and adopted.

Other regulatory bodies consider SOPs for investigators a requirement (Health Canada).

1.1.5 GCP Applicability

Good Clinical Practice applies to the three main parties involved in a clinical trial: (1) the sponsor of the clinical investigation, (2) the principal investigator (PI), and (3) the Institutional Review Board (IRB) or Ethic Review Board or Committee (see Figure 1.1)

In the case where the principal investigator initiates the clinical trial (academic clinical trials not sponsored by industry), he/she also bears the responsibilities of the sponsor. This is procedurally defined as a dual role sponsor – investigator. The dual role is discussed in-depth later to allow institutions that foster this type of human research to understand the scope of FDA regulatory applicability.

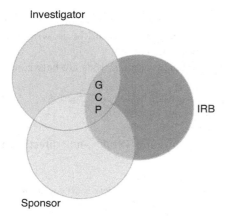

Figure 1.1   Parties in a clinical trial.

The role and responsibilities of the clinical research sponsor are discussed first since the sponsor is the initiator of a clinical study.

1.2 ROLE OF THE SPONSOR OF A CLINICAL INVESTIGATION

The **sponsor** of a clinical trial is an individual, corporation, manufacturer, agency, or scientific institution that assumes the sponsor's responsibilities as described in Good Clinical Practice and the applicable regulatory requirements. For FDA purposes, the sponsor is the individual or company that identifies himself or itself as such in Form 1571[2].

1.2.1 GCP: Responsibilities of a Sponsor of a Clinical Trial

When a sponsor initiates the development of an investigational product in humans, he/she assumes the following responsibilities:

1. *Provide for Quality Assurance (QA) and Quality Control (QC).* The clinical trial sponsor has to confirm and demonstrate that all clinical trial activities are conducted in accordance with GCP and regulatory requirements.
   The sponsor should:
   (a) *Implement QA and QC.* The sponsor is responsible for implementing and maintaining quality assurance (audit capabilities) and quality control (monitoring clinical trials) systems with written SOPs to ensure that trials are conducted and data are generated, documented (recorded), and reported in compliance with the protocol, GCP, and the applicable regulatory requirement(s).
   (b) *Secure Agreements with Parties.* The sponsor is responsible for securing agreement from all involved parties to ensure direct access to all trial-related sites, source data/documents, and reports for the purpose of monitoring and auditing by the sponsor, and inspection by domestic and foreign regulatory authorities.
   Agreements, made by the sponsor with the investigator/institution and any other parties involved with the clinical trial, should be in writing as part of the protocol or in a separate agreement.
   The potential agreements within parties in clinical trials are between:
   • Sponsor – investigator
   • Sponsor–contract research organization/third party contractors
   • Sponsor– clinical trial laboratory testing facility
   • Investigator – institution
   • Investigator– site management organization (SMO—not directly included in GCP or regulations)

---

[2]Form 1571—FDA Investigational New Drug Application. Available at http://www.fda.gov/downloads/AboutFDA/ReportsManualForms/Forms/UCM083533.pdf.

Site management organizations are identified as new players in the clinical research industry, providing services to the investigator site as coordinators and other clinical trial site-specific services. Note that these organizations, new in the clinical research setting, are not mentioned yet in GCP or regulatory requirements, and therefore are not subject to regulatory inspections. It is very important to address that, although SMOs are necessarily not inspected by the regulator, the sponsor should inspect the SMO that provides services for the investigator's site and determine that it is fully compliant with GCP and regulations. Also, the sponsor has to know in detail the agreement between the investigator site and the SMO to guarantee accessibility to records and quality of the activity contracted.

(c) *Provide for Monitoring*. Quality control should be applied to each stage of data handling to ensure that all data are reliable and have been processed correctly.

2. *Hire a Contract Research Organization (CRO)*. In the last two decades, the industry faced an increased number of clinical trials and locations of investigational sites. Also, with the adoption of GCP and the increase in regulatory demands, sponsors had to seek out third party service providers for clinical research activities to remain compliant and to complete projects in a timely manner. GCP is very clear on the relationship between a sponsor and a sponsor's service provider.

(a) *Transfer Trial-Related Duties*. A sponsor may transfer any or all of the sponsor's trial-related duties and functions to a CRO, but the ultimate responsibility for the quality and integrity of the trial data always resides with the sponsor. Any trial-related duty and function that is transferred to and assumed by a CRO should be specified in writing. **The transfer should be done in writing in the format of a contract agreement where the transferred duties must be detailed.** Any trial-related duties and functions not specifically transferred to and assumed by a CRO are retained by the sponsor.

Transfer of duties does not mean in any case transfer of responsibilities. Note that the sponsor is always ultimately responsible for the quality and integrity of the trial data.

(b) *Ensure QA and QC of CRO*. The CRO should implement quality assurance and quality control. CRO compliance to GCP and regulatory requirements is the same as for the sponsor; therefore, it has to implement QA and QC.

(c) *CRO Shares Sponsor's Responsibilities*. All references to a sponsor in GCP also apply to a CRO to the extent that a CRO has assumed the trial-related duties and functions of a sponsor, and therefore assumes responsibility for the activities contracted.

3. *Provide for Medical Expertise*. Clinical trials, although not a replacement for medical treatment, have to always consider the health, safety, and well-being

of the subjects involved. Medical decisions on efficacy and/or safety have to be done in an ongoing manner from the part of a sponsor of a clinical study. Therefore, the sponsor should designate appropriately qualified medical personnel who will be readily available to advise on trial-related medical questions or problems. Since it may become impractical for a company/sponsor to keep on staff full-time medical experts, then, if necessary, outside consultant(s) may be appointed for this purpose.

4. *Develop Trial Design.* The design of the clinical trial is the sponsor's responsibility. The sponsor should utilize qualified individuals (e.g., biostatisticians, clinical pharmacologists, and physicians) as appropriate, throughout all stages of the trial process, from designing the Protocol and Case Report Forms and planning the analyses to analyzing and preparing interim and final clinical trial reports.

5. *Provide for Trial Management, Data Handling, and Recordkeeping.*

   (a) *Clinical Trial Management Personnel Qualifications.* Adequately qualified personnel are the key to a successful study. The sponsor should utilize appropriately qualified individuals to supervise the overall conduct of the trial, to handle the data, to verify the data, to conduct the statistical analyses, and to prepare the trial reports.

   (b) *Independent Data Monitoring Committee.* Due to the complexity and size of clinical trials, continuous safety surveillance of the subjects has to be provided to ensure that the sponsor reacts to safety concerns appropriately. The sponsor should consider establishing an independent data monitoring committee (IDMC) to assess the progress of a clinical trial, including the safety data and the critical efficacy endpoints at intervals, and to recommend to the sponsor whether to continue, modify, or stop a trial. The IDMC should have written operating procedures and should maintain written records of all its meetings.

   (c) *Electronic Data.* GCP established the grounds for many aspects of data management when electronic systems are utilized; nevertheless, regulators defined specific requirements that are to be implemented strictly to assure compliance.

   When using electronic trial data handling and/or remote electronic trial data systems, the sponsor should:

   (i) **Perform System Validation.** Ensure and document that the electronic data processing system(s) conforms to the sponsor's established requirements for completeness, accuracy, reliability, and consistent intended performance (i.e., validation).

   (ii) **Use Standard Operating Procedures.** Maintain SOPs for using these systems.

   (iii) **Institute an Audit Trail.** Ensure that the systems are designed to permit data changes in such a way that the data changes are documented and that there is no deletion of entered data (i.e., maintain an audit trail, data trail, edit trail).

(iv) *Provide System Security.* Maintain a security system that prevents unauthorized access to the data.

(v) *Determine Access Privileges.* Maintain a list of the individuals who are authorized to make data changes.

(vi) *Provide for Data Backup.* Maintain adequate backup of the data.

(d) *Blinding.* Maintaining the blinding in a clinical trial is essential to reduce bias on the observations on the part of the blinded parties. The sponsor should safeguard the blinding, if any (e.g., maintain the blinding during data entry and processing).

(e) *Source Data.* Source data should exist for all information collected in a clinical trial CRF. If data are transformed during processing, it should always be possible to compare the original data and observations with the processed data. The sponsor should ensure access to the source at any time.

(f) *Unique Subject Code.* The sponsor should use an unambiguous subject identification code that allows identification of all the data reported for each subject. Also, since we should have one code for a subject, we should have one subject for a code. In other words, we cannot re-enroll subjects who previously participated in the study(ies) without particular exemptions (extensions, open label phases, etc.) since they are not going to contribute with new data, and long or repeated exposure to the investigational product may be of a higher unknown risk.

1.2.2 Essential Documents for the Clinical Trial

GCP states that "the sponsor, or other owners of the data, should retain all of the sponsor-specific essential documents pertaining to the trial." The sponsor should have an organized system, the Trial Master File (TMF) for filing, searching, and retrieving those essential documents. The sponsor also should maintain an electronic Trial Master File that contains all the essential documents for the clinical trial either electronically generated or scanned from the original paper documents. Accessibility privileges and all other assurances for the integrity of the filing system should follow the criteria for electronic systems in clinical trials. Also, the sponsor must keep the original paper documents as a source.

Retention of the Essential Documents for the Clinical Trial   The sponsor should retain all sponsor-specific essential documents in conformance with the applicable regulatory requirement(s) of the country(ies) where the product is approved, and/or where the sponsor intends to apply for approval(s).

Archiving of the Essential Documents for the Clinical Trial After Discontinuation of Development   If the sponsor discontinues the clinical development of an investigational product (i.e., for any or all indications, routes of administration, or dosage forms), the sponsor should maintain all sponsor-specific essential documents for at least 2 years after formal discontinuation or in conformance with the applicable regulatory requirement(s) (in Canada the record retention is for 25 years).

Notification   If the sponsor discontinues the clinical development of an investigational product, the sponsor should notify all the trial investigators/institutions and all the regulatory authorities.

Transfer of Data Ownership   In these times when mergers and acquisitions of pharmaceutical and biotech companies occur frequently, it is important that there is evidence of ownership of (and responsibility for) the data for the investigational products that continue development. Transferring data ownership also entitles the transfer of sponsors' responsibilities before the eyes of the regulator. GCP states that "any transfer of ownership of the data should be reported to the appropriate authority(ies), as required by the applicable regulatory requirement(s)."

Records Retention   Access to records by the parties of a clinical study will allow the regulator through compliance inspections, to confirm the adherence to requirements. A comparison with original records at the investigator site and at the sponsor's site will only be possible if the records are retained for a minimum established period. The sponsor-specific essential documents should be retained until at least 2 years after the last approval of a marketing application in an ICH region and until there are no pending or contemplated marketing applications in an ICH region or at least 2 years have elapsed since the formal discontinuation of clinical development of the investigational product. These documents should be retained for a longer period, however, if required by the applicable regulatory requirement(s) or if needed by the sponsor (in Canada the record retention is for 25 years).

Also, the sponsor should inform the investigator(s)/institution(s) in writing of the need for record retention (e.g., in the clinical trial agreement) and should notify the investigator(s)/institution(s) in writing when the trial-related records are no longer needed. The sponsor is responsible for ensuring access to source documents and other clinical trial documents at the investigator site to auditors and regulatory inspectors for the stipulated period of time.

1.2.3   Investigator Selection

Clinical trial success depends on selecting the right investigator with the right resources and facilities. The selection process should be detailed in procedures that are very explicit on the sponsor's selection criteria.

GCP establishes that the sponsor is responsible for selecting the investigator(s)/institution(s).

Investigator's Qualifications   GCP states that "each investigator should be qualified by training and experience." It is very important to note that the investigator is responsible for the medical care of subjects; therefore, when selecting an investigator, he/she should be qualified and able to provide that medical care (licensed to practice in the province, state, or region), and at the same time be able to conduct the study at the site.

Resources at the Investigator's Site   The investigator should have personnel to assist him/her in the undertaking of a clinical trial since it entails various activities that are time consuming and extensive. The investigator must comply with GCP, regulatory requirements, and specific study requirements at all times, and a person who acts as a coordinator for those activities may be required. Also, the investigator site should have, if required by the protocol, a study nurse and co/subinvestigators who will have certain responsibilities delegated to them in order to achieve the study's objectives in a timely and compliant manner. GCP states that "the investigator should have adequate resources to properly conduct the trial for which he/she is selected." If organization of a coordinating committee is to be achieved and/or selection of coordinating investigator(s) is to be done in multicenter trials, their organization and/or selection are the sponsor's responsibilities.

Protocol and Investigator's Brochure   The sponsor has the responsibility to write and have the protocol and Investigator's Brochure available for the investigator to peruse before committing to the study.

GCP states that "before entering an agreement with an investigator/institution to conduct a trial, the sponsor should provide the investigator(s)/institution(s) with the protocol and an up-to-date Investigator's Brochure, and should provide sufficient time for the investigator/institution to review the protocol and the information provided."

Agreement with the Investigator/Institution   It is essential that the sponsor secure a written agreement with the investigator/institution before the clinical trial is initiated.

The sponsor should obtain the investigator's/institution's agreement for the following: (1) to conduct the trial in compliance with GCP, with the applicable regulatory requirement(s), and with the protocol agreed to by the sponsor and given approval/favorable opinion by the IRB/IEC; (2) to comply with procedures for data recording/reporting; (3) to permit monitoring, auditing, and inspection; and (4) to retain the trial-related essential documents until the sponsor informs the investigator/institution that these documents are no longer needed.

The sponsor and the investigator/institution should sign the protocol, or an alternative document, to confirm this agreement.

Although GCP states the four essential elements of compliance in the agreement between an investigator and sponsor (compliance to regulatory requirements and GCP and IRB approved protocol; compliance to protocol procedures for data recording/reporting; permitting monitoring and audit; and document retention), it is important to emphasize that the sponsor should include specific conditions for the implementation of the clinical trial at the site and consequences for violations, deviations, or noncompliant activities.

1.2.4 Allocation of Responsibilities

GCP states that, prior to initiating a trial, the sponsor should define, establish, and allocate all trial-related duties and functions. This activity is usually performed by the assigned project manager/project leader, who, with the guide of the protocol and the Investigator's Brochure, will estimate and allocate clinical trial functions to ensure compliance and project control.

1.2.5 Compensation to Subjects and Investigators

Compensation to Subjects for Trial-Related Injuries A subject compensation clause is applicable when regulatory authorities establish that requirement and when the patient is financially responsible for his/her medical care. It is essential that this issue is discussed properly in the patient information and consent form. GCP establishes that "if required by the applicable regulatory requirement(s), the sponsor should provide insurance or should indemnify (legal and financial coverage) the investigator/institution against claims arising from the trial — compensation for trial related injuries — except for claims that arise from malpractice and/or negligence."

It is important to note that any claims that arise from malpractice and/or negligence against the site are the investigator's responsibility and he/she should have knowledge of that to make sure his/her professional insurance covers clinical trial situations. In the same way, the sponsors are responsible for their part in any claim.

GCP states that "the sponsor's policies and procedures (SOPs) should address the costs of treatment of trial subjects in the event of trial-related injuries in accordance with the applicable regulatory requirement(s)."

Other Types of Compensation to Trial Subjects It is generally accepted that healthy volunteers who participate in Phase I studies be compensated for their participation in the study. However, depending on the regulatory body, patients in Phase II or III trials might not be entitled to monetary compensation. It is important to note that the compensation should not be construed as a benefit. The GCP guidance states that "when trial subjects receive compensation, the method and manner of compensation should comply with applicable regulatory requirement(s)."

1.2.6 Financing

Previously, we discussed the GCP guideline where there should be a written agreement between the sponsor and the investigator on the compliance terms of the clinical study — the Clinical Trial Agreement (CTA). Also, the sponsor and the investigator must agree on the financial terms of the study. Those financial terms can be part of the CTA, but not necessarily. The parties may have an independent financial agreement that also has to be available for inspection. GCP states in this matter that "the financial aspects of the trial should be documented in an agreement between the sponsor and the investigator/institution."

It is important to note that investigations of a site within an institution may be subject to institutional overhead. Financial agreements between the sponsor and investigator will set the basis for the amount of overhead charged.

1.2.7 Notification/Submission to Regulatory Authorities

Drugs, biologicals, and medical devices intended to be tested in humans are regulated products. Sponsors must ensure that they request and obtain regulatory authorization to start the development of an investigational product in humans. The scope of the regulated product may vary from country to country, but the applicability of the principle is the same.

The GCP principle states that "before initiating the clinical trial(s), the sponsor (or the sponsor and the investigator, if required by the applicable regulatory requirement(s)) should submit any required application(s) to the appropriate authority(ies) for review, acceptance, and/or permission (as required by the applicable regulatory requirement(s)) to begin the trial(s). Any notification/submission should be dated and contain sufficient information to identify the protocol."

1.2.8 Confirmation of Review by IRB/IEC

The sponsor does not communicate with the IRB/IEC directly. However, in a January 2010 draft guidance, the FDA suggested that the sponsor should submit annual safety reports directly to IRBs since they have access to a broader base of information. All communications and interactions within the IRB/IEC are done through the investigator.

According to GCP regarding IRB/IEC, it is the sponsor's responsibility to obtain the following from the investigator/institution:

- *IRB/IEC Identification.* The name and address of the investigator's/institution's IRB/IEC.
- *IRB/IEC Compliance Statement.* A statement obtained from the IRB/IEC that it is organized and operates according to GCP and the applicable laws and regulations.
- *IRB/IEC Approval Document of the Clinical Trial Documents.* Documented IRB/IEC approval/favorable opinion and, if requested by the sponsor, a current copy of protocol, written informed consent form(s), and any other written information to be provided to subjects, subject recruiting procedures, and documents related to payments and compensation available to the subjects, and any other documents that the IRB/IEC may have requested.
- *Protocol Amendments Approvals.* If the IRB/IEC conditions its approval/favorable opinion upon change(s) in any aspect of the trial, such as modification(s) of the protocol, written informed consent form and any other written information to be provided to subjects, and/or other procedures, the sponsor should obtain from the investigator/institution a copy of the modification(s) made and the date approval/favorable opinion was given by the IRB/IEC.
- *Continuous IRB/IEC Review and Approval.* The sponsor should obtain from the investigator/institution documentation and dates of any IRB/IEC reapprovals/reevaluations with favorable opinion, and of any withdrawals or suspensions of approval/favorable opinion.

1.2.9   Information on Investigational Products

This part refers to the sponsor's responsibility to have a complete preclinical development dossier that will support the application to develop the investigational product in humans, and to write and update an Investigator's Brochure.

GCP states that "when planning trials, the sponsor should ensure that sufficient safety and efficacy data from nonclinical studies and/or clinical trials are available to support human exposure by the route, at the dosages, for the duration, and in the trial population to be studied."

Safety and efficacy information together with the risk assessment of the investigational product will eventually change as development evolves. It is important to reassess risk as new data becomes available and inform the investigator and the patient if that information is relevant.

GCP states that "the sponsor should update the Investigator's Brochure as significant new information becomes available."

1.2.10   Manufacturing, Packaging, Labelling, and Coding Investigational Products

Characterization, Manufacturing, and Labeling of the Investigational Product   The sponsor should ensure that the investigational product(s) (including active comparator(s) and placebo, if applicable) is characterized as appropriate to the stage of development of the product(s), is manufactured in accordance with any applicable GMP, and is coded and labeled in a manner that protects the blinding, if applicable. In addition, the labeling should comply with applicable regulatory requirement(s).

Storage Conditions   The sponsor should determine, for the investigational product(s), acceptable storage temperatures, storage conditions (e.g., protection from light), storage times, reconstitution fluids and procedures, and devices for product infusion, if any. The sponsor should inform all involved parties (e.g., monitors, investigators, pharmacists, storage managers) of these determinations.

Packaging of the Investigational Product   Investigational products are shipped and stored and therefore handled before being provided to the eligible subjects. The investigational product(s) should be packaged to prevent contamination and unacceptable deterioration during transport and storage.

Coding and Decoding of the Investigational Product   In clinical trials that are designed to be blinded to reduce bias in data collection and reporting, the process to access the identification of the blinded product is called **Decoding**. Decoding procedures should be followed in case of patient emergency as stated in the protocol. The decoding procedure and the unblinding of a patient investigational product should not compromise the blinding of the study. Decoding is performed through the use of code breakers that are paper format or electronic. Access to codebreakers should be 24/7. Any decoding, including involuntary decoding, should be properly documented.

GCP states that "in blinded trials, the coding system for the investigational product(s) should include a mechanism that permits rapid identification of the product(s) in case of a medical emergency, but does not permit undetectable breaks of the blinding."

Investigational Product Changes and Bioequivalence Studies   "If significant formulation changes are made in the investigational or comparator product(s) during the course of clinical development, the results of any additional studies of the formulated product(s) (e.g., stability, dissolution rate, bioavailability) needed to assess whether these changes would significantly alter the pharmacokinetic profile of the product should be available prior to the use of the new formulation in clinical trials."

1.2.11   Supplying and Handling Investigational Products

The sponsor has the responsibility to supply investigational product to the investigational site (investigator/institution) in a timely manner and in compliance with GCP and regulatory requirements.

Supply   The sponsor should not supply an investigator/institution with the investigational product(s) until the sponsor obtains all required documentation (e.g., approval/favorable opinion from IRB/IEC and regulatory authority(ies)).

Procedures for Investigational Product Handling   The sponsor should ensure that written procedures include instructions that the investigator/institution should follow for the handling and storage of investigational product(s) for the trial and documentation thereof. The procedures should address adequate and safe (1) receipt, (2) handling, (3) storage, (4) dispensing, (5) retrieval of unused product from subjects, and (6) return of unused investigational product(s) to the sponsor (or alternative disposition if authorized by the sponsor and in compliance with the applicable regulatory requirement(s)).

Investigational Product Records   The sponsor should provide and maintain records for the handling of the investigational product. The sponsor should maintain records that document (1) shipment, (2) receipt, (3) disposition, (4) return, and (5) destruction of the investigational product(s).

Investigational Product Retrieval or Recall   The sponsor should maintain a system for retrieving investigational products and documenting this retrieval (e.g., for deficient product recall, reclaim after trial completion, expired product reclaim).

Investigational Product Disposition   The sponsor should maintain a system for the disposition of unused investigational product(s) and for the documentation of this disposition. That system should be explained in the protocol and followed by the investigator.

Investigational Product Stability   Ongoing stability testing will ensure that the investigational product remains stable during the clinical trial. GCP states that "the sponsor should take steps to ensure that the investigational product(s) are stable over the period of use."

Investigational Product Samples   The sponsor should maintain sufficient quantities of the investigational product(s) used in the trials to reconfirm specifications, should this become necessary, and maintain records of batch sample analyses and characteristics. To the extent stability permits, samples should be retained either until the analyses of the trial data are complete or as required by the applicable regulatory requirement(s), whichever represents the longer retention period.

1.2.12   Record Access

Access to records should be available at any time to source verify data entered in the Case Report Forms, to audit for compliance, and to allow access to regulatory inspectors.

GCP states that "the sponsor should ensure that it is specified in the protocol or other written agreement that the investigator(s)/institution(s) provide direct access to source data/documents for trial-related monitoring, audits, IRB/IEC review, and regulatory inspection."

Verification of Patient Consent to Record Access   The sponsor should verify that each subject has consented, in writing, to direct access to his/her original medical records for trial-related monitoring, audit, IRB/IEC review, and regulatory inspection.

1.2.13   Safety Information

As principles of the Declaration of Helsinki, it is important that the sponsor ensures patient safety and well-being at all times. The risk and benefit assessment of an investigational product is started when the sponsor initially submits the request for authorization to regulatory authorities to run the first clinical trial in humans.

However, safety is of concern at all times, and the sponsor is responsible for the ongoing safety evaluation of the investigational product(s).

Safety Issues   Any unexpected and serious adverse event, if confirmed, may affect adversely the safety of the subjects in a study.

Communication of Safety Issues   GCP states that "the sponsor should promptly notify all concerned investigator(s)/institution(s) and the regulatory authority(ies) of findings that could:

- affect adversely the safety of subjects,
- impact the conduct of the trial, or
- alter the IRB/IEC's approval/favorable opinion to continue the trial."

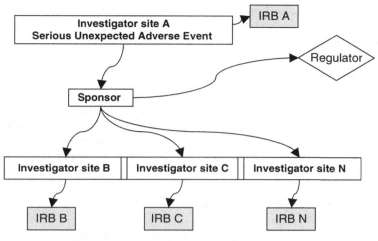

Figure 1.2   SAE reporting flow chart.

1.2.14   Adverse Drug Reaction Reporting

Serious Unexpected Adverse Drug Reactions   These reactions are serious in nature and severity and never previously reported in the Investigator's Brochure or any other safety record. Those reactions may affect the risk–benefit assessment and therefore should be communicated immediately. The sponsor must report them as soon as it becomes aware of the event, following GCP and regulatory requirements.

The sponsor should expedite the reporting to all concerned investigator(s)/institution(s), to the IRB(s)/IEC(s), where required, and to the regulatory authority(ies) of all adverse drug reactions (ADRs) that are both serious and unexpected. (see Figure 1.2.)

SAE Reporting Compliance   SAE reporting process and timeliness should comply with (1) applicable regulatory requirement(s) and (2) ICH Guideline for Clinical Safety Data Management: Definitions and Standards for Expedited Reporting.

Safety Updates and Periodic Reports   This reporting is in addition to the serious adverse event reporting and clinical trials reports. GCP stipulates that "the sponsor should submit to the regulatory authority(ies) all safety updates and periodic reports, as required by applicable regulatory requirement(s)." This reporting should be mostly generated by the Independent Data Monitoring Committee or Data Safety Monitoring Boards appointed by the sponsor and who have the responsibility to follow all safety issues for the investigational product in question and conduct an ongoing safety assessment.

1.2.15   Monitoring

The monitoring of a clinical trial is a sponsor responsibility and should be conducted periodically to confirm patient safety and data quality. One of the biggest issues facing the sponsor is to determine how often is often enough. Sponsors should have SOPs that very clearly and concisely describe the process and frequency of monitoring clinical trials.

Monitoring of a clinical trial is a sponsor's responsibility.

Purposes: GCP states that the purposes of trial monitoring are to verify that (1) the rights and well-being of **human subjects** are protected; (2) the reported trial **data** are accurate, complete, and verifiable from source documents; and (3) the conduct of the trial is in **compliance** with the currently approved protocol/amendment(s), with GCP, and with the applicable regulatory requirement(s).

Selection and Qualifications of Monitors

Selection of Monitors   The sponsor appoints the monitors of a study. Although there are no specifics to the relationship between the monitor and the sponsor, he/she can be either a full-time employee of the sponsor, a contractor, or a CRO.

Background and Qualifications of Monitors   GCP indicates that "monitors should be appropriately trained, and should have the scientific and/or clinical knowledge needed to monitor the trial adequately. A monitor's qualifications should be documented." Mostly, a monitor can be a person with a degree in science, nursing, medicine, or other health-related discipline.

Clinical Trials Specific Training and Education   Besides the required background, GCP states that "monitors should be thoroughly familiar with the investigational product(s), the protocol, written informed consent form and any other written information to be provided to subjects, the sponsor's SOPs, GCP, and the applicable regulatory requirement(s)." Having internal full-time monitors allows the sponsor to thoroughly train and instruct them on the company's SOPs and protocol requirements, although having contractors or CROs performing monitoring activities will accelerate resource-wise the study completion.

Extent and Nature of Monitoring   GCP indicates that the sponsor should ensure that the trials are adequately monitored. However, there is no indication on what is considered adequate, leaving it up to the sponsor to determine, according to the protocol design, resources, and compliance procedures, the frequency and extent of monitoring for a clinical trial site.

The guidance also states that "the sponsor should determine the appropriate extent and nature of monitoring. The determination of the extent and nature of monitoring should be based on considerations such as the objective, purpose, design, complexity, blinding, size, and endpoints of the trial." To comply with this the sponsor should have SOPs that detail the process for estimating and allocating monitoring capabilities as well as monitoring procedures and reporting.

Monitoring Strategies   There are some common strategies that have been accepted and utilized in the last several years by sponsors of clinical trials:

- On-site monitoring (most common and accepted)
- Central monitoring (fax, email, web based)
- Statistically controlled sampling of data monitoring

GCP specifies that "in general there is a need for on-site monitoring, before, during, and after the trial; however, in exceptional circumstances the sponsor may determine that central monitoring in conjunction with procedures such as investigators' training and meetings, and extensive written guidance can assure appropriate conduct of the trial in accordance with GCP. Statistically controlled sampling may be an acceptable method for selecting the data to be verified."

Monitor's Responsibilities   The monitor's responsibilities are defined by the scope of the compliance requirements to oversee all clinical trial activities at the investigator site.

GCP details that "the monitor(s) in accordance with the sponsor's requirements should ensure that the trial is conducted and documented properly by carrying out the following activities when relevant and necessary to the trial and the trial site."

1. ***Communication Link with Site***: The monitor acts as the main line of communication between the sponsor and the investigator. The monitor is the eyes and ears of the sponsor and the link between the investigator site and the sponsor. Also, during monitoring visits the monitor has to verify the documentation and products as described below.

2. ***Investigator Site Qualifications, Resources, and Facilities***. Verifying that the investigator has adequate qualifications and resources and they remain adequate throughout the trial period; that facilities, including laboratories, equipment, and staff, are adequate to safely and properly conduct the trial and remain adequate throughout the trial period.

3. ***Investigational Product(s)***

   (a) *Storage*. Storage times and conditions of the investigational product(s) are acceptable, and supplies are sufficient throughout the trial.

   (b) *Supply*. The investigational product(s) are supplied only to subjects who are eligible to receive it and at the protocol specified dose(s).

   (c) *Instructions for Use*. Subjects are provided with necessary instruction on properly using, handling, storing, and returning the investigational product(s).

   (d) *Accountability*. The receipt, use, and return of the investigational product(s) at the trial sites are controlled and documented adequately.

   (e) *Drug Disposition*. The disposition of unused investigational product(s) at the trial sites complies with applicable regulatory requirement(s) and is in accordance with the sponsor.

4. *Protocol Adherence*. Verifying that the investigator follows the approved protocol and all approved amendment(s), if any.

5. *Informed Consent*. Verifying that written informed consent was obtained before each subject's participation in the trial.

6. *Up-to-Date Version of Investigator's Brochure, Documents, and Trial Supplies*. Ensuring that the investigator receives the current Investigator's Brochure, all documents, and all trial supplies needed to conduct the trial properly and to comply with the applicable regulatory requirement(s).

7. *Training of Investigator Site*. Ensuring that the investigator and the investigator's trial staff are adequately informed about the trial.

8. *Protocol and Clinical Trial Agreement Compliance*. Verifying that the investigator and the investigator's trial staff are performing the specified trial functions, in accordance with the protocol and any other written agreement between the sponsor and the investigator/institution, and have not delegated these functions to unauthorized individuals.

9. *Patient Eligibility*. Verifying that the investigator is enrolling only eligible subjects.

10. *Subject Recruitment Rate*. The monitor has to report the subject recruitment rate.

11. *Source Data Availability*. Verifying that source documents and other trial records are accurate, complete, up-to-date, and well maintained.

12. *Investigator Reports*. Verifying that the investigator provides all the required reports, notifications, applications, and submissions, and that these documents are accurate, complete, timely, legible, dated, and identify the trial.

13. *Source Data Verification*. Checking the accuracy and completeness of the CRF entries, source documents, and other trial-related records against each other. The monitor specifically should verify the following:

(a) *Data*. The data required by the protocol are reported accurately on the CRFs and are consistent with the source documents.

(b) *Therapy*. Any dose and/or therapy modifications are well documented for each of the trial subjects.

(c) *Safety*. Adverse events, concomitant medications, and intercurrent illnesses are reported in accordance with the protocol on the CRFs.

(d) *Patient Visit Compliance*. Visits that the subjects fail to make, tests that are not conducted, and examinations that are not performed are clearly reported as such on the CRFs.

(e) *Withdrawals/Dropouts*. All withdrawals and dropouts of enrolled subjects from the trial are reported and explained on the CRFs.

(f) *Error Capture and Resoultion*. The investigator is informed of any CRF entry error, omission, or illegibility. The monitor should ensure that appropriate corrections, additions, or deletions are made, dated, explained (if necessary), and initialed by the investigator or by a member of the investigator's trial staff who is authorized to initial CRF changes for the investigator. This authorization should be documented.

(g) *Adverse Event Reporting.* Determining whether all adverse events (AEs) are appropriately reported within the time periods required by GCP, the protocol, the IRB/IEC, the sponsor, and the applicable regulatory requirement(s).

(h) *Essential Documents.* Determining whether the investigator is maintaining the essential documents

(i) *Protocol Deviations.* Communicating deviations from the protocol, SOPs, GCP, and the applicable regulatory requirements to the investigator and taking appropriate action designed to prevent recurrence of the detected deviations.

Monitoring Procedures   Although specific procedures are not defined in GCP guidelines, the sponsor should establish (1) the SOPs on monitoring clinical trial sites to achieve full compliance, and (2) that the monitor adheres to those procedures as well as study-specific monitoring requirements.

Monitoring Report   The monitoring report is a clinical trial document that must be generated at the end of each monitoring visit to a site. This document will evidence the visit and status of the site. A copy of the document must remain in the Trail Master File. The investigator, although not provided with a copy, should be informed in the form of a letter or other communication tool of the findings to the site. A visit is also considered a phone contact, email, or other type of communication with the site where trial-specific issues were discussed. The monitoring report should be provided to the monitor in the form of a template with all specific GCP/regulatory compliance requirements.

GCP recommends the following regarding a monitoring visit:

- *Written Report*: The monitor should submit a written report to the sponsor after each trial-site visit or trial-related communication.

- *Contents of the Report.* Reports should include the date, site, name of the monitor, and name of the investigator or other individual(s) contacted. Reports should include a summary of what the monitor reviewed and the monitor's statements concerning the significant findings/facts, deviations and deficiencies, conclusions, actions taken or to be taken, and/or actions recommended to secure compliance.

- *Report Review.* The review and follow-up of the monitoring report with the sponsor should be documented by the sponsor's designated representative.

1.2.16   AUDIT

The sponsor is required to implement a quality management system that will allow internal quality assurance inspections to confirm compliance to SOPs, GCPs, and regulatory requirements.

GCP requires that the sponsor performs quality inspections considering the following principles.

- *Independence.* The site/sponsor auditors (QA) must be independent from clinical operations (QC monitoring) and that independence must be established in the company's SOPs.

- *Evaluation.* The main objective of an internal audit is to evaluate the trial conduct, compliance with the protocol, company's SOPs, and adherence to GCPs and regulatory requirements.

Selection and Qualifications of Auditors   Auditors or internal inspectors are employed by the sponsor to perform internal quality assurance functions that will ensure compliance. The sponsor should make certain that (1) inspectors are independent from clinical functions (QC) and (2) the auditors are qualified by training, and experience to conduct audits properly. All auditor qualifications should be documented in the form of background, training, and certifications.

Auditing Procedures   The sponsor should have, within the quality management system, SOPs on:

- Clinical trial audit scope (what to audit)
- Clinical trial audit procedure (how to conduct an audit)
- Clinical trial audit frequency (how often to audit)
- Clinical trial audit reporting (how to report findings)

Site Selection Criteria for Inspection   Also, the sponsor should have criteria for selecting sites/trials for audit. Those criteria should be based on the GCP criteria as follows:

- *Submission Priorty.* Trials should be selected according to the importance of the trial in the submissions to regulatory authorities

- *Subject Number.* Trials that provide most of the safety and efficacy data, because they enrolled the most patients, should be audited.

- *Type of Study.* Pivotal studies provide most of the safety end efficacy data due to design and size.

- *Complexity of Trial.* Studies with a high degree of complexity should be inspected for adherence to the protocol.

- *Risk to Subject.* Studies that involve a higher risk to subjects should be inspected to verify that patient safety was not compromised at any point.

- *Problems Identified in Previous Inspections.* Studies conducted at sites that had problems in prior inspections should be reinspected to verify that remedial procedures were implemented.

Reporting of Findings

- All the noncompliant activities should be documented by the auditor in writing and copies should be obtained of necessary supporting documents.
- The audit report should be a confidential document, and the regulatory authorities should not request a copy as GCP requires one "to maintain the independence and value of the audit function."
- There are two cases where the regulator can seek access to QA inspection reports: (1) If the quality assurance systems per se appear not to be compliant to GCP/regulatory requirements due to serious findings by authorities, or (2) during legal proceedings.

Audit Certificate   The audit certificate is a document that confirms, when filed in the sponsor's Trial Master File, that a GCP quality audit has been conducted at a particular site.

GCP states that "when required by applicable law or regulation, the sponsor should provide an audit certificate."

1.2.17   Noncompliance

It is the sponsor's responsibility to identify and remediate SOP, GCP, and regulatory noncompliant activities (see Figure 1.3).

Any serious or persistent noncompliant activity or violation deserves termination of the investigator site and notification to regulatory authorities.

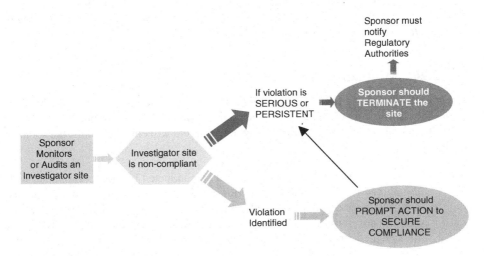

Figure 1.3   Noncompliance.

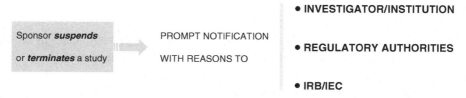

Figure 1.4   Termination or suspension of a trial.

1.2.18   Premature Termination or Suspension of a Trial

Termination or suspension of a study has many implications, especially to a patient's safety. Upon the sponsor's decision to terminate or suspend a study, the investigator/institution, regulatory authorities, and IRB/IEC should be notified promptly, stating the reasons. (see Figure 1.4.)

1.2.19   Clinical Trial/Study Reports

- *Responsibility*. The sponsor bears the responsibility of writing the Clinical Trial Report in the format required by the regulatory authorities.
- *Submission*. Every written report must be submitted to the regulatory authorities.
- *Trial Data*. Every clinical trial must have documented the results in a Clinical Trial Report.
- *Report Completion*. The report must be written for completed and for prematurely terminated studies.
- *Marketing Applications*: For marketing applications, the report must meet either the standards of the *ICH Guideline for Structure and Content of Clinical Study Reports* or country specific regulatory requirements.

1.2.20   Multicenter Trials

Drug development in the pharmaceutical industry has increased in complexity. The design of protocols includes centers located nationally or internationally to achieve enrollment in shorter times. Since many investigators will enroll patients, the sponsor must ensure the following:

- *Protocol Adherence*. The study should be conducted in strict compliance with the agreed protocol that was previously approved, if required, by regulatory authorities, and given approval/favorable opinion by the IRB/IEC. If every investigator introduces changes or deviates from the protocol, the study cannot be analyzed since the number of variables introduced becomes unknown, the safety of patients becomes compromised, and the study would not represent the objectives of the protocol.

- *Data Collection.* Data is going to be collected in Case Report Forms (CRFs). All investigators will collect data in preestablished CRFs. Supplemental CRFs should be provided for investigators who provide additional data.

- *Management of Study Investigators.* GCPs states that "the responsibilities of coordinating investigator(s) and the other participating investigators are documented prior to the start of the trial."

- *Investigators' Guidance.* All investigators should be given instructions on (1) following the protocol, (2) complying with a uniform set of standards for the assessment of clinical and laboratory findings, and (3) completing the CRFs.

- *Investigators' Interaction.* GCP states that "communication between investigators is facilitated." It is very important that the sponsor ensures that the communication does not compromise the blinding of the study (if blinded) or promote bias in patient assessments.

1.3 ROLE OF THE INSTITUTIONAL REVIEW BOARD/INDEPENDENT ETHICS COMMITTEE (IRB/IEC)

1.3.1 Responsibilities

Ethics review of research involving human subjects is a requirement stated in the Declaration of Helsinki.

The Institutional Review Board or Independent Ethics Committee has the mandate to safeguard the **Rights, Safety**, and **Well-being** of all trial subjects. GCP notes that "special attention should be paid to trials that may include vulnerable subjects." Subjects like children, the elderly, or patients with mental limitations cannot provide consent and are considered vulnerable.

The IRB/IEC should perform the following *activities* for *ethics review*.[3]

Document Gathering The following documents should be collected by the IRB/IEC before reviewing a proposed study:

- Trial protocol(s)/amendment(s)
- Written informed consent form(s) and consent form updates that the investigator proposes for use in the trial
- Subject recruitment procedures (e.g., advertisements)
- Written information to be provided to subjects (the Informed Consent Form template)
- Investigator's Brochure (IB)
- Available safety information
- Information about payments and compensation available to subjects

[3]Information Sheets. Guidance for Institutional Review Boards and Clinical Investigators. 1998 Update—A Self-Evalution Checklist for IRBs can be found at http://www.fda.gov/ScienceResearch/SpecialTopics/RunningClinicalTrials/GuidanceInformationSheetsandNotices/ucm118063.htm.

- The investigator's current curriculum vitae and/or other documentation evidencing qualifications
- Any other documents that the IRB/IEC may need to fulfill its responsibilities

Review of Documentation   GCP states that the IRB/IEC should:

- **Review** a proposed clinical trial within a *reasonable time*;
- **Document** its views in writing, clearly identifying the trial, the documents reviewed, and the dates; and
- **Issue a Decision** on the conduct of the trial for the investigator site with (1) an approval/favorable opinion; (2) modifications required prior to its approval/favorable opinion; (3) disapproval/negative opinion; and (4) termination/suspension of any prior approval/favorable opinion (if deemed necessary in the light of new information regarding safety and compliance).

1.3.2   Considerations for Review

- *Investigator's Qualifications.* As documented by a current curriculum vitae and/or by any other relevant documentation the IRB/IEC requests.
- *Continuous Review.* The IRB/IEC should conduct a continuous review of each ongoing trial (to assess safety and ethics issues in a continuous manner), or at least once a year or depending on the degree of risk to subjects.

1.3.3   Additional Information to be Provided To Subjects

The IRB/IEC may request additional information to be given to subjects when, in the judgment of the IRB/IEC, that information would add meaningfully to the protection of the rights, safety, and/or well-being of the subjects.

Nontherapeutic Trials   When subjects who provided consent through legally acceptable representatives are enrolled in nontherapeutic trials (where no benefits can be expected to a subject, as in a bioequivalence study), the IRB/IEC has to determine if the proposed protocol and/or other documentation adequately addresses relevant ethical concerns and is compliant with regulations.

Emergency Situations   When a study is designed to take place in an emergency setting, the design of the study and the protocol has to indicate that, in the case when consent is not possible directly from the subject or legally appointed representative, the IRB/IEC should determine if the proposed protocol and/or other document(s) adequately addresses relevant ethical concerns and meets applicable regulatory requirements for such trials. This GCP guideline should be applied carefully in conjunction with regulatory requirements. Note that this type of study may affect the population at large within the investigator site, and public consultation may be further needed to address specifically this ethical issue.

Payment to Study Subjects   Payment to study subjects is a fact, although it remains controversial as to the amount and conditions of payment. To address any possible ethical issue, the IRB/IEC should review the following:

- Amount of payment to subjects
- Method of payment to subjects
        This review should provide assurance that it does not represent coercion or undue influence on the trial subjects.
        The method of payment should be **prorated** and **unconditional**. Prorated means proportional to the subject's participation. This is to avoid a subject remaining in a study with the sole purpose of collecting money. If a subject remains in a study just to collect payment and an adverse event develops, that may mean unnecessary exposure to an unsafe product if the subject remains for financial reasons. Unconditional means not wholly contingent on completion of the trial by the subject.

Payment Information in the Consent Form   To avoid misunderstandings regarding financial compensation to study subjects, GCP determines that "the IRB/IEC should ensure that information regarding payment to subjects, including the methods, amounts, and schedule of payment to trial subjects, is set forth in the written informed consent form and any other written information to be provided to subjects. The way payment is prorated should be specified."

Composition, Functions, and Operations

1. **Reasonable Number of Members.** GCP states that the IRB/IEC should consist of a reasonable number of members, who collectively have the qualifications and experience to review and evaluate the science, medical aspects, and ethics of the proposed trial. It is recommended that the IRB/IEC should include (a) at least five members, (b) at least one member whose primary area of interest is in a nonscientific area, and (c) at least one member who is independent of the institution/trial site.

2. **Independence of the Members.** Only those IRB/IEC members who are **independent of the investigator and the sponsor** of the trial should vote/provide opinion on a trial-related matter. The issue of the investigator sitting on an IRB/IEC is resolved as GCP states that "the investigator may provide information on any aspect of the trial, but should not participate in the deliberations of the IRB/IEC or in the vote/opinion of the IRB/IEC." That must be documented clearly in the minutes of the meeting. The other issue is having the sponsor hold an IRB/IEC within the family of companies that decides on its own studies. That scenario has to be evaluated in detail since employees of the sponsor cannot sit and deliberate on a study without being in conflict of interest.

3. **Membership.** A list of IRB/IEC members and their qualifications should be maintained. That list should be available to the investigator, the sponsor, and the regulator upon request.

4. **Function According to Standard Operating Procedures.** The IRB/IEC should perform its functions according to written operating procedures, should maintain written records of its activities and minutes of its meetings, and should comply with GCP and with the applicable regulatory requirement(s).

5. **Decission with Quorum.** An IRB/IEC should make its decisions at announced meetings at which at least a quorum, as stipulated in its written operating procedures, is present.

6. **Voting Privileges.** Only members who participate in the IRB/IEC review and discussion should vote/provide their opinion and/or advise.

7. **Nonmembers.** An IRB/IEC may invite nonmembers with expertise in special areas for assistance.

IRB/IEC Standard Operating Procedures   The IRB/IEC should establish, document in writing, and follow its procedures.

SOPs required as in GCP guidelines

1. **Composition.** An SOP determining its composition (names and qualifications of the members) and the authority under which it is established.

2. **Meeting Schedulling.** An SOP on the scheduling process for IRB/IEC meetings.

3. **Member Notification of Meetings.** An SOP on methods of notifying its members of a meeting.

4. **Meeting Conduct.** An SOP on how the IRB/IEC meetings should be conducted.

5. **Initial and Continuous Review.** An SOP to determine the process for the initial and continuous review of a trial.

6. **Frequency of Review.** An SOP to determine the frequency of continuing review of a trial, as appropriate.

7. **Expedited Review.** SOPs that determine the process for expedited review and approval/favorable opinion of minor change(s) in ongoing trials that have the approval/favorable opinion of the IRB/IEC.

8. **Enrolment Dependent on IRB/IEC Approval.** An SOP that specifies that no subject should be admitted to a trial before the IRB/IEC issues its written approval/favorable opinion of the trial. *Admission to a trial means that a subject signed consent and is going to provide either data or take active investigational product under a protocol.*

9. **Protocol Deviations**. The IRB/IEC should have procedures specifying that no deviations from, or changes of, the protocol should be initiated without prior written IRB/IEC approval/favorable opinion of an appropriate amendment, **except (a) when necessary to eliminate immediate hazards to the subjects or (b) when the change(s) involves only logistical or administrative aspects of the trial** (e.g., change of monitor(s), telephone number(s)).

10. **Investigators Reporting.** An SOP specifying that the investigator should promptly report the following to the IRB/IEC:

    (a) *Deviations.* Deviations from, or changes of, the protocol to eliminate immediate hazards to the trial subjects.

    (b) *Changes.* Changes in the protocol or information in the safety data increasing the risk to subjects and/or affecting significantly the conduct of the trial.

    (c) *Adverse Drug Reactions.* All adverse drug reactions (ADRs) **that are** both **serious** and **unexpected.**

    (d) *New Information.* Any new information that may affect adversely the safety of the subjects or the conduct of the trial.

11. **IRB/IEC Notifications.** The IRB/IEC should have SOPs to ensure that the investigator/institution notified promptly and in writing concerning (a) its trial-related decisions/opinions, (b) The reasons for its decisions/opinions, and (c) procedures for appeal of its decisions/opinions.

Records   It is very important to demonstrate compliance to the regulator. Therefore, the IRB/IEC should provide records of their activities. The GCP establishes that "the IRB/IEC should retain all relevant records" as, for example, written procedures, membership lists, lists of occupations/affiliations of members, submitted documents by the investigator, minutes of meetings (complete and appropriate), and correspondence (with the investigators) for a period of at least 3 years after completion of the trial and make them available upon request from the regulatory authority(ies).

The IRB/IEC may be asked by investigators, sponsors, or regulatory authorities to provide its written procedures and membership lists.

1.4   ROLES AND RESPONSIBILITIES OF THE CLINICAL TRIAL INVESTIGATOR

The clinical trial investigator is responsible for the clinical trial at the site and has to comply with GCP and regulatory requirements in an extent that demonstrates that patient safety and data integrity is assured.

GCP establishes several requirements for compliance that are going to be the basis for essential aspects of a regulatory inspection.

1.4.1   Investigator's Qualifications and Agreements

- *Qualifications.* The investigator(s) should be qualified by education, training, and experience to assume responsibility for the proper conduct of the trial; should meet all the qualifications specified by the applicable regulatory requirement(s); and should provide evidence of such qualifications through up-to-date curriculum vitae and/or other relevant documentation requested by the sponsor, the IRB/IEC, and/or the regulatory authority(ies).

- *Training in Use of the Investigational Product.* The investigator should be thoroughly familiar with the appropriate use of the investigational product(s), as described in the protocol, in the current Investigator's Brochure, in the product information, and in other information sources provided by the sponsor.

- *GCP and Regualtory Compliance.* The investigator should be aware of, and should comply with, GCP and the applicable regulatory requirements.

- *Monitring and Inspection.* The investigator/institution should permit monitoring and auditing by the sponsor, and inspection by the appropriate regulatory authority(ies).

- *Clinical Trial Personnel List.* The investigator should maintain a list of appropriately qualified persons to whom the investigator has delegated significant trial-related duties.

1.4.2   Adequate Resources

The following are considered resources in a clinical trial:

- *Prospective Subjects.* The investigator should be able to demonstrate (e.g., based on retrospective data) a potential for recruiting the required number of suitable subjects within the agreed upon recruitment period.

- *Time to Conduct the Study.* The investigator should have sufficient time to properly conduct and complete the trial within the agreed upon trial period.

- *Qualified Personnel.* The investigator should have available an adequate number of qualified staff and adequate facilities for the foreseen duration of the trial to conduct the trial properly and safely.

- *Training of Personnel.* The investigator should ensure that all persons assisting with the trial are adequately informed about the protocol, the investigational product(s), and their trial-related duties and functions.

1.4.3   Medical Care of Trial Subjects

The Declaration of Helsinki considers that the duty of a clinical investigator is foremost the medical care of the subjects involved.

- *Medical Decission in a Trial.* A qualified physician (or dentist, when appropriate), who is an investigator or a subinvestigator for the trial, should be responsible for all trial-related medical (or dental) decisions.

- *Medical Care After Adverse Event.* During and following a subject's participation in a trial, the investigator/institution should ensure that adequate medical care is provided to a subject for any adverse events, including clinically significant laboratory values, related to the trial. The investigator/institution should inform a subject when medical care is needed for intercurrent illness(es) of which the investigator becomes aware.

- *Communication with Primary Physician.* It is recommended that the investigator inform the subject's primary physician about the subject's participation in the trial if the subject has a primary physician and if the subject agrees to the primary physician being informed.

- *Reason for Subject Withdrawal.* Although a subject is not obliged to give his/her reason(s) for withdrawing prematurely from a trial, the investigator should make a reasonable effort to ascertain the reason(s), while fully respecting the subject's rights. This point is very important because the reasons for withdrawal may be unreported adverse events or lack of efficacy, which, for private reasons, the subject may not wish to share with the study personnel. These outcomes are very important for the conclusion of the study.

1.4.4 Communication with IRB/IEC

The investigator is the party in a clinical trial who communicates directly with the IRB/IEC. Therefore, the investigator is responsible for the following activities:

- *Obtain Written Approval/Favorable Opinion for the Protocol.* Before initiating a trial, the investigator/institution should have written and dated approval/favorable opinion from the IRB/IEC for the trial protocol, written informed consent forms consent form updates, subject recruitment procedures (e.g., advertisements), and any other written information to be provided to subjects.

- *Provide IRB/IEC with Investigator's Brochure.* As part of the investigator's/institution's written application to the IRB/IEC, the investigator/institution should provide the IRB/IEC with a current copy of the Investigator's Brochure. If the Investigator's Brochure is updated during the trial, the investigator/institution should supply a copy of the updated Investigator's Brochure to the IRB/IEC.

- *Continuous Submission of Documents.* During the trial the investigator/institution should provide to the IRB/IEC all documents subject to review.

1.4.5 Compliance with Protocol

- *Conduct Study in Compliance with Protocol.* (1) The investigator/institution should conduct the trial in compliance with the protocol agreed to by the sponsor and, if required, (2) by the regulatory authority(ies), and (3) which was given approval/favorable opinion by the IRB/IEC.

- *Confirmation of Agreement.* The investigator/institution and the sponsor should sign the protocol, or an alternative contract, to confirm agreement.

- *Protocol Deviations.*

    (1) *Implementation.* The investigator should not implement any deviation from, or changes of, the protocol without agreement by the sponsor and prior review and documented approval/favorable opinion from the IRB/IEC of an amendment, **except** (a) where necessary to eliminate immediate hazard(s) to trial subjects, or (b) when the change(s) involves only logistical or administrative aspects of the trial (e.g., change in monitor(s), change of telephone number(s)).

    (2) *Documentation.* The investigator, or person designated by the investigator, should document and explain any deviation from the approved protocol.

    (3) *Communication.* As described previously, the investigator may implement a deviation from, or a change of, the protocol to eliminate immediate hazard(s) to trial subjects without prior IRB/IEC approval/favorable opinion. Following the implemented deviation or change, the reasons for it, and, if appropriate, the proposed protocol amendment(s) should be submitted (a) to the IRB/IEC for review and approval/favorable opinion (after the fact), (b) to the sponsor for agreement and, if required, (c) to the regulatory authority(ies).

1.4.6 Investigational Product(s)

The sponsor is responsible for providing the investigational product, and the investigator bears the responsibility to store, dispense, and account for the investigational product according to the protocol at the trial site.

GCP requires the following from the investigator:

- *Accountability.* Responsibility for investigational product(s) accountability at the trial site(s) rests with the investigator/institution.

- *Delegate Accountability to Pharmacist.* Where allowed/required, the investigator/institution may/should assign some or all of the investigator's/institution's duties for investigational product(s) accountability at the trial site(s) to an appropriate pharmacist or another appropriate individual who is under the supervision of the investigator/institution.

- *Recordkeeping.* The investigator/institution and/or a pharmacist or other appropriate individual, who is designated by the investigator/institution, should maintain records of the **product's delivery** to the trial site, the inventory at the site, the use by each subject, **and the return** to the sponsor or **alternative disposition of unused product(s).** These records should include dates, quantities, batch/serial numbers, expiration dates (if applicable), and the unique code numbers assigned to the investigational product(s) and trial subjects. Investigators should maintain records that document adequately that the subjects were provided the doses specified by the protocol and reconcile all investigational product(s) received from the sponsor.

- *Storage.* The investigational product(s) should be stored as specified by the sponsor and in accordance with applicable regulatory requirement(s).

- *Use Controlled.* The investigator should ensure that the investigational product(s) are used only in accordance with the approved protocol.

- *Subject Instruction and Follow-up.* The investigator, or a person designated by the investigator/institution, should explain the correct use of the investigational product(s) to each subject and should check, at intervals appropriate for the trial, that each subject is following the instructions properly.

1.4.7   Randomization Procedures and Unblinding

Randomization of treatment groups as well as blinding are performed to ensure an equitable number of subjects are exposed to a particular treatment arm and that data is collected in an unbiased manner. Therefore, the investigator has the responsibility to follow randomization procedures and keep the blinding in the study, if applicable.

GCP states that the investigator should (1) follow the trial's randomization procedures, if any; (2) ensure that the code is broken only in accordance with the protocol, and (3) if the trial is blinded, the investigator should promptly document and explain to the sponsor any premature unblinding (e.g., accidental unblinding, unblinding due to a serious adverse event) of the investigational product(s).

1.4.8   Informed Consent of Trial Subjects

The investigator bears the responsibility for obtaining consent from subjects before any clinical trial procedure or data collection for trial purposes is initiated.

The consent process has to be followed and documented according to regulatory requirements.

GCP requires the following:

- *Compliance.* In obtaining and documenting informed consent, the investigator should comply with the applicable regulatory requirement(s) and should adhere to GCP and to the ethical principles that have their origin in the Declaration of Helsinki.

- *IRB/IEC Approval.* Prior to the beginning of the trial, the investigator should have the IRB/IEC's written approval/favorable opinion of the written informed consent form and any other written information to be provided to subjects.

- *Revision.* The written informed consent form and any other written information to be provided to subjects should be revised whenever important new information becomes available that may be relevant to the subject's consent. Any revised written informed consent form and written information should receive the IRB/IEC's approval/favorable opinion in advance of use.

- *Reconsent of Subjects.* The subject or the subject's legally acceptable representative should be informed in a timely manner if new information becomes available that may be relevant to the subject's willingness to continue participation in the trial. The communication of this information should be documented.

- *No Coercion.* Neither the investigator, nor the trial staff, should coerce or unduly influence a subject to participate or to continue to participate in a trial.

- *No Release of Liability.* None of the oral and written information concerning the trial, including the written informed consent form, should contain any language that causes the subject or the subject's legally acceptable representative to waive or to appear to waive any legal rights, or that releases or appears to release the investigator, the institution, the sponsor, or their agents from liability for negligence.

- *Subject Fully Informed.* The investigator, or a person designated by the investigator, should fully inform the subject or, if the subject is unable to provide informed consent, the subject's legally acceptable representative, of all pertinent aspects of the trial including the written information and the approval/favorable opinion by the IRB/IEC.

- *Language.* The language used in the oral and written information about the trial, including the written informed consent form, should be as nontechnical as practical and should be understandable to the subject or the subject's legally acceptable representative and the impartial witness, where applicable.

- *Time to Decide.* Before informed consent may be obtained, the investigator, or a person designated by the investigator, should provide the subject or the subject's legally acceptable representative with ample time and opportunity to enquire about details of the trial and to decide whether or not to participate in the trial. All questions about the trial should be answered to the satisfaction of the subject or the subject's legally acceptable representative.

- *Signature Prior to Participation.* Prior to a subject's participation in the trial, the written informed consent form should be signed and personally dated by the subject or by the subject's legally acceptable representative, and by the person who conducted the informed consent discussion.

- *Witness.* If a subject is unable to read or if a legally acceptable representative is unable to read, an impartial witness should be present during the entire informed consent discussion. After the written informed consent form, and any other written information to be provided to subjects, is read and explained to the subject or the subject's legally acceptable representative, and after the subject or the subject's legally acceptable representative has orally consented to the subject's participation in the trial and, if capable of doing so, has signed and personally dated the informed consent form, the witness should sign and personally date the consent form. By signing the consent form, the witness attests that the information in the consent form and any other written information was accurately explained to, and apparently understood by, the subject or the subject's legally acceptable representative, and that informed consent was freely given by the subject or the subject's legally acceptable representative.

- *Elements of the Informed Consent Form.* Both the informed consent discussion and the written informed consent form and any other written information to be provided to subjects should include explanations of the following:

1. That the trial involves research.
2. The purpose of the trial.
3. The trial treatment(s) and the probability for random assignment to each treatment.
4. The trial procedures to be followed, including all invasive procedures.
5. The subject's responsibilities.
6. Those aspects of the trial that are experimental.
7. The reasonably foreseeable risks or inconveniences to the subject and, when applicable, to an embryo, fetus, or nursing infant.
8. The reasonably expected benefits. When there is no intended clinical benefit to the subject, the subject should be made aware of this.
9. The alternative procedure(s) or course(s) of treatment that may be available to the subject, and their important potential benefits and risks.
10. The compensation and/or treatment available to the subject in the event of trial-related injury.
11. The anticipated prorated payment, if any, to the subject for participating in the trial.
12. The anticipated expenses, if any, to the subject for participating in the trial.
13. That the subject's participation in the trial is voluntary and that the subject may refuse to participate or may withdraw from the trial, at any time, without penalty or loss of benefits to which the subject is otherwise entitled.
14. The monitor(s), the auditor(s), the IRB/IEC, and the regulatory authority(ies) will be granted direct access to the subject's original medical records for verification of clinical trial procedures and/or data, without violating the confidentiality of the subject, to the extent permitted by the applicable laws and regulations and that, by signing a written informed consent form, the subject or the subject's legally acceptable representative is authorizing such access.
15. Records identifying the subject will be kept confidential and, to the extent permitted by the applicable laws and/or regulations, will not be made publicly available. If the results of the trial are published, the subject's identity will remain confidential.
16. That the subject or the subject's legally acceptable representative will be informed in a timely manner if information becomes available that may be relevant to the subject's willingness to continue participation in the trial.
17. The person(s) to contact for further information regarding the trial and the rights of trial subjects, and whom to contact in the event of trial-related injury.
18. The foreseeable circumstances and/or reasons under which the subject's participation in the trial may be terminated.

19. The expected duration of the subject's participation in the trial.

20. The approximate number of subjects involved in the trial.

- *Copy of Signed Consent.* Prior to participation in the trial, the subject or the subject's legally acceptable representative should receive a copy of the signed and dated written informed consent form and any other written information provided to the subjects. During a subject's participation in the trial, the subject or the subject's legally acceptable representative should receive a copy of the signed and dated consent form updates and a copy of any amendments to the written information provided to subjects.

- *Consent Through Legal Representative.* When a clinical trial (therapeutic or nontherapeutic) includes subjects who can only be enrolled in the trial with the consent of the subject's legally acceptable representative (e.g., minors or patients with severe dementia), the subject should be informed about the trial to the extent compatible with the subject's understanding and, if capable, the subject should sign and personally date the written informed consent.

- *Nontherapeutic Trials.* Except as described above, a nontherapeutic trial (i.e., a trial in which there is no anticipated direct clinical benefit to the subject), should be conducted in subjects who personally give consent and who sign and date the written informed consent form.

- *Conditions for Nontherapeutic Trials.* Nontherapeutic trials may be conducted in subjects with consent of a legally acceptable representative provided the following conditions are fulfilled:

  1. The objectives of the trial cannot be met by means of a trial in subjects who can give informed consent personally.

  2. The foreseeable risks to the subjects are low.

  3. The negative impact on the subject's well-being is minimized and low.

  4. The trial is not prohibited by law.

  5. The approval/favorable opinion of the IRB/IEC is expressly sought on the inclusion of such subjects, and the written approval/favorable opinion covers this aspect. Such trials, unless an exception is justified, should be conducted in patients having a disease or condition for which the investigational product is intended. Subjects in these trials should be particularly closely monitored and should be withdrawn if they appear to be unduly distressed.

  6. In emergency situations, when prior consent of the subject is not possible, the consent of the subject's legally acceptable representative, if present, should be requested. When prior consent of the subject is not possible, and the subject's legally acceptable representative is not available, enrollment of the subject should require measures described in the protocol and/or elsewhere, with documented approval/favorable opinion by the IRB/IEC, to protect the rights, safety, and well-being of the subject and to ensure compliance with applicable regulatory requirements. The subject or the subject's legally acceptable representative should be informed about the trial as soon as possible and consent to continue and other consent as appropriate should be requested.

1.4.9   Records and Reports

Proper documentation in clinical trials is very important to demonstrate compliance with and adherence to regulatory requirements. The investigator may be required to generate specific reports to document clinical trial activities and collect data for the sponsor. The following are the GCP requirements for records and reports:

- *Accuracy, Completeness, Legibility, and Timeliness of the Data Reported.* The investigator should ensure the accuracy, completeness, legibility, and timeliness of the data reported to the sponsor in the CRFs and in all required reports (any delays may compromise the safety of patients).
- *Source Data.* Data reported on the CRF, which are derived from source documents, should be consistent with the source documents or the discrepancies should be explained.
- *Data Correction or Resolution.* Any change or correction to a CRF should be dated, initialed, and explained (if necessary) and should not obscure the original entry (i.e., an audit trail should be maintained); this applies to both written and electronic changes or corrections. Sponsors should provide guidance to investigators and/or the investigators' designated representatives on making such corrections. Sponsors should have written procedures to assure that changes or corrections in CRFs made by the sponsor's designated representatives are documented, are necessary, and are endorsed by the investigator. The investigator should retain records of the changes and corrections. Note that no changes to data are allowed if not authorized by the investigator.
- *Record Retention.* The investigator/institution should maintain the trial documents as specified in Essential Documents for the Conduct of a Clinical Trial (see table Essential Documents for the Conduct of a Clinical Trial part 8 of the ICH/GCP guideline) and as required by the applicable regulatory requirement(s). The investigator/institution should take measures to prevent accidental or premature destruction of these documents.
- *Retention Times.* Essential documents should be retained until at least 2 years after the last approval of a marketing application in an ICH region and until there are no pending or contemplated marketing applications in an ICH region or at least 2 years have elapsed since the formal discontinuation of clinical development of the investigational product. These documents should be retained for a longer period, however, if required by the applicable regulatory requirements (e.g., in Canada it is 25 years) or by an agreement with the sponsor. It is the responsibility of the sponsor to inform the investigator/institution as to when these documents are no longer need to be retained.
- *Financial Agreements.* The financial aspects of the trial should be documented in an agreement between the sponsor and the investigator/institution.
- *Access to Records.* Upon request of the monitor, auditor, IRB/IEC, or regulatory authority, the investigator/institution should make available for direct access all requested trial-related records.

1.4.10 Progress Reports

The investigator may need to provide progress reports to the sponsor and to the IRB/IEC from time to time to update the safety and enrollment status.

1. The investigator should submit written summaries of the trial status to the IRB/IEC annually, or more frequently, if requested by the IRB/IEC.

2. The investigator should promptly provide written reports to the sponsor, the IRB/IEC, and, where applicable, the institution on any changes significantly affecting the conduct of the trial and/or increasing the risk to subjects.

Safety Reporting

1. All serious adverse events (SAEs) (Unexpected) should be reported immediately to the sponsor except for those SAEs that the protocol or other document (e.g., Investigator's Brochure) identifies as not needing immediate reporting. The immediate reports should be followed promptly by detailed, written reports. The immediate and follow-up reports should identify subjects by unique code numbers assigned to the trial subjects rather than by the subjects' names, personal identification numbers, and/or addresses. The investigator should also comply with the applicable regulatory requirement(s) related to the reporting of unexpected serious adverse drug reactions to the regulatory authority(ies) and the IRB/IEC.

2. Adverse events and/or laboratory abnormalities identified in the protocol as critical to safety evaluations should be reported to the sponsor according to the reporting requirements and within the time periods specified by the sponsor in the protocol.

3. For reported deaths, the investigator should supply the sponsor and the IRB/IEC with any additional requested information (e.g., autopsy reports and terminal medical reports).

1.4.11 Premature Termination or Suspension of a Trial

If the trial is prematurely terminated or suspended for any reason, the investigator/institution should promptly inform the trial subjects, should assure appropriate therapy and follow-up for the subjects, and, where required by the applicable regulatory requirement(s), should inform the regulatory authority(ies). In addition:

1. If the investigator terminates or suspends a trial without prior agreement of the sponsor (a) the investigator should inform the institution where applicable, and (b) the investigator/institution should promptly inform the sponsor and the IRB/IEC, and should provide the sponsor and the IRB/IEC with a detailed written explanation of the termination or suspension.

2. If the sponsor terminates or suspends a trial (a) the investigator should promptly inform the institution where applicable, and (b) the investigator/institution should promptly inform the IRB/IEC and provide the IRB/IEC with a detailed written explanation of the termination or suspension.

3. If the IRB/IEC terminates or suspends its approval/favorable opinion of a trial, (a) the investigator should inform the institution where applicable, and (b) the investigator/institution should promptly notify the sponsor and provide the sponsor with a detailed written explanation of the termination or suspension.

4. Upon completion of the trial, the investigator, where applicable, should inform the institution; the investigator/institution should provide the IRB/IEC with a summary of the trial's outcome and the regulatory authority(ies) with any reports required.

1.5 CLINICAL TRIAL PROTOCOL AND PROTOCOL AMENDMENTS

The contents of a trial protocol should generally include the following topics. However, site-specific information may be provided on separate protocol page(s), or addressed in a separate agreement, and some of the information listed below may be contained in other protocol referenced documents, such as an Investigator's Brochure.

1.5.1 Contents of Trial Protocol

1. *General Information*

    (a) Protocol title, protocol identifying number, and date. Any amendment(s) should also bear the amendment number(s) and date(s).

    (b) Name and address of the sponsor and monitor (if other than the sponsor).

    (c) Name and title of the person(s) authorized to sign the protocol and the protocol amendment(s) for the sponsor.

    (d) Name, title, address, and telephone number(s) of the sponsor's medical expert (or dentist when appropriate) for the trial.

    (e) Name and title of the investigator(s) who is (are) responsible for conducting the trial, and the address and telephone number(s) of the trial site(s).

    (f) Name, title, address, and telephone number(s) of the qualified physician (or dentist, if applicable), who is responsible for all trial-site related medical (or dental) decisions (if other than investigator).

    (g) Name(s) and address(es) of the clinical laboratory(ies) and other medical and/or technical department(s) and/or institutions involved in the trial.

2. *Background Information*

    (a) Name and description of the investigational product(s).

    (b) A summary of findings from nonclinical studies, that potentially have clinical significance, and from clinical trials that are relevant to the trial.

    (c) Summary of the known and potential risks and benefits, if any, to human subjects.

(d) Description of and justification for the route of administration, dosage, dosage regimen, and treatment period(s).

(e) A statement that the trial will be conducted in compliance with the protocol, GCP, and the applicable regulatory requirement(s).

(f) Description of the population to be studied.

(g) References to literature and data that are relevant to the trial and that provide background for the trial.

3. *Trial Objectives and Purpose.* A detailed description of the objectives and the purpose of the trial.

4. *Trial Design.* The scientific integrity of the trial and the credibility of the data from the trial depend substantially on the trial design. A description of the trial design, should include the following:

(a) A specific statement of the primary endpoints and the secondary endpoints, if any, to be measured during the trial.

(b) A description of the type/design of trial to be conducted (e.g., double-blind, placebo-controlled, parallel design) and a schematic diagram of trial design, procedures, and stages.

(c) A description of the measures taken to minimize/avoid bias, including (i) randomization and (ii) blinding.

(d) A description of the trial treatment(s) and the dosage and dosage regimen of the investigational product(s). Also include a description of the dosage form, packaging, and labeling of the investigational product(s).

(e) The expected duration of subject participation, and a description of the sequence and duration of all trial periods, including follow-up, if any.

(f) A description of the "stopping rules" or "discontinuation criteria" for individual subjects, parts of trial, and entire trial.

(g) Accountability procedures for the investigational product(s), including the placebo(s) and comparator(s), if any.

(h) Maintenance of trial treatment randomization codes and procedures for breaking codes.

(i) The identification of any data to be recorded directly on the CRFs (i.e., no prior written or electronic record of data), and considered source data.

5. *Selection and Withdrawal of Subjects*

(a) Subject inclusion criteria.

(b) Subject exclusion criteria.

(c) Subject withdrawal criteria (i.e., terminating investigational product treatment/trial treatment) and procedures specifying (i) when and how to withdraw subjects from the trial/investigational product treatment; (ii) the type and timing of the data to be collected for withdrawn subjects; (iii) whether and how subjects are to be replaced; and (iv) the follow-up for subjects withdrawn from investigational product treatment/trial treatment.

6. *Treatment of Subjects*

   (a) The treatment(s) to be administered, including the name(s) of all the product(s), the dose(s), the dosing schedule(s), the route/mode(s) of administration, and the treatment period(s), including the follow-up period(s) for subjects for each investigational product treatment/trial treatment group/arm of the trial.

   (b) Medication(s)/treatment(s) permitted (including rescue medication) and not permitted before and/or during the trial.

   (c) Procedures for monitoring subject compliance.

7. *Assessment of Efficacy*

   (a) Specification of the efficacy parameters.

   (b) Methods and timing for assessing, recording, and analyzing efficacy parameters.

8. *Assessment of Safety*

   (a) Specification of safety parameters.

   (b) The methods and timing for assessing, recording, and analyzing safety parameters.

   (c) Procedures for eliciting reports of and for recording and reporting adverse events and intercurrent illnesses.

   (d) The type and duration of the follow-up of subjects after adverse events.

9. *Statistics*

   (a) A description of the statistical methods to be employed, including timing of any planned interim analysis(ses).

   (b) The number of subjects planned to be enrolled. In multicenter trials, the numbers of enrolled subjects projected for each trial site should be specified. Reason for choice of sample size, including reflections on (or calculations of) the power of the trial and clinical justification, should be given.

   (c) The level of significance to be used.

   (d) Criteria for the termination of the trial.

   (e) Procedure for accounting for missing, unused, and spurious data.

   (f) Procedures for reporting any deviation(s) from the original statistical plan (any deviation(s) from the original statistical plan should be described and justified in the protocol and/or in the final report, as appropriate).

   (g) The selection of subjects to be included in the analyses (e.g., all randomized subjects, all dosed subjects, all eligible subjects, evaluable subjects).

10. *Direct Access to Source Data/Documents.* The sponsor should ensure that it is specified in the protocol or other written agreement that the investigator(s)/institution(s) will permit trial-related monitoring, audits, IRB/IEC review, and regulatory inspection(s), providing direct access to source data/documents.

11. *Quality Control and Quality Assurance*

12. *Ethics*. Description of ethical considerations relating to the trial.

13. *Data Handling and Recordkeeping*

14. *Financing and Insurance*. Financing and insurance if not addressed in a separate agreement.

15. *Publication Policy*. Publication policy, if not addressed in a separate agreement.

16. *Supplements*

1.5.2   Investigator's Brochure

Introduction   The Investigator's Brochure (IB) is a compilation of the clinical and nonclinical data on the investigational product(s) that are relevant to the study of the product(s) in human subjects. Its purpose is to provide investigators and others involved in the trial with information to facilitate their understanding of the rationale for, and their compliance with, many key features of the protocol, such as the dose, dose frequency/interval, methods of administration, and safety monitoring procedures. The IB also provides insight for the clinical management of study subjects during the course of the clinical trial. The information should be presented in a concise, simple, objective, balanced, and nonpromotional form that enables a clinician, or potential investigator, to understand it and make his/her own unbiased risk–benefit assessment of the appropriateness of the proposed trial. For this reason, a medically qualified person should generally participate in the editing of an IB, but the contents of the IB should be approved by the disciplines that generated the described data.

The GCP guideline delineates the minimum information that should be included in an IB and provides suggestions for its layout. It is expected that the type and extent of information available will vary with the stage of development of the investigational product. If the investigational product is marketed and its pharmacology is widely understood by medical practitioners, an extensive IB may not be necessary. Where permitted by regulatory authorities, a basic product information brochure, package leaflet, or labeling may be an appropriate alternative, provided that it includes current, comprehensive, and detailed information on all aspects of the investigational product that might be of importance to the investigator. If a marketed product is being studied for a new use (i.e., a new indication), an IB specific to that new use should be prepared. The IB should be reviewed at least annually and revised as necessary in compliance with a sponsor's written procedures. More frequent revision may be appropriate, depending on the stage of development and the generation of relevant new information. However, in accordance with Good Clinical Practice, relevant new information may be so important that it should be communicated to the investigators, and possibly to the Institutional Review Boards (IRBs)/Independent Ethics Committees (IECs) and/or regulatory authorities before it is included in a revised IB.

Generally, the sponsor is responsible for ensuring that an up-to-date IB is made available to investigators and the investigators are responsible for providing the up-to-date IB to the responsible IRBs/IECs. In the case of an investigator-sponsored trial, the sponsor–investigator should determine whether a brochure is available from the commercial manufacturer. If the investigational product is provided by the sponsor–investigator, then he/she should provide the necessary information to the trial personnel. In cases where preparation of a formal IB is impractical, the sponsor–investigator should provide, as a substitute, an expanded background information section in the trial protocol that contains the minimum current information described in the guideline.

General Considerations   The IB should include:

1. *Title Page.* This should provide the sponsor's name, the identity of each investigational product (i.e., research number, chemical or approved generic name, and trade name(s) where legally permissible and desired by the sponsor), and the release date. It is also suggested that an edition number, and a reference to the number and date of the edition it supersedes, be provided.

2. *Confidentiality Statement.* The sponsor may wish to include a statement instructing the investigator/recipients to treat the IB as a confidential document for the sole information and use of the investigator's team and the IRB/IEC.

Contents of the Investigator's Brochure   The IB should contain the following sections, each with literature references where appropriate:

1. *Table of Contents*

2. *Summary.* A brief summary (preferably not exceeding two pages) should be given, highlighting the significant physical, chemical, pharmaceutical, pharmacological, toxicological, pharmacokinetic, metabolic, and clinical information available that is relevant to the stage of clinical development of the investigational product.

3. *Introduction.* A brief introductory statement should be provided that contains the chemical name (and generic and trade name(s) when approved) of the investigational product(s), all active ingredients, the investigational product(s) pharmacological class and its expected position within this class (e.g., advantages), the rationale for performing research with the investigational product(s), and the anticipated prophylactic, therapeutic, or diagnostic indication(s). Finally, the introductory statement should provide the general approach to be followed in evaluating the investigational product.

4. *Physical, Chemical, and Pharmaceutical Properties and Formulation.* A description should be provided of the investigational product substance(s) (including the chemical and/or structural formula(s)), and a brief summary should be given of the relevant physical, chemical, and pharmaceutical properties.

   To permit appropriate safety measures to be taken during the course of the trial, a description of the formulation(s) to be used, including excipients, should be provided and justified if clinically relevant. Instructions for the storage and handling of the dosage form(s) should also be given.

   Any structural similarities to other known compounds should be mentioned.

5. *Nonclinical Studies.* The results of all relevant nonclinical pharmacology, toxicology, pharmacokinetic, and investigational product metabolism studies should be provided in summary form. This summary should address the

methodology used, the results, and a discussion of the relevance of the findings to the investigated therapeutic and the possible unfavorable and unintended effects in humans.

The information provided may include the following, as appropriate, if known/available:

(a) Species tested

(b) Number and sex of animals in each group

(c) Unit dose (e.g., milligram/kilogram (mg/kg))

(d) Dose interval

(e) Route of administration

(f) Duration of dosing

(g) Information on systemic distribution

(h) Duration of postexposure follow-up

(i) Results, including nature and frequency of pharmacological or toxic effects, severity or intensity of pharmacological or toxic effects, time to onset of effects, reversibility of effects, duration of effects, dose response

Tabular format/listings should be used whenever possible to enhance the clarity of the presentation.

The following sections should discuss the most important findings from the studies, including the dose response of observed effects, the relevance to humans, and any aspects to be studied in humans. If applicable, the effective and nontoxic dose findings in the same animal species should be compared (i.e., the therapeutic index should be discussed). The relevance of this information to the proposed human dosing should be addressed. Whenever possible, comparisons should be made in terms of blood/tissue levels rather than on a mg/kg basis.

(a) *Nonclinical Pharmacology.* A summary of the pharmacological aspects of the investigational product and, where appropriate, its significant metabolites studied in animals, should be included. Such a summary should incorporate studies that assess potential therapeutic activity (e.g., efficacy models, receptor binding, and specificity) as well as those that assess safety (e.g., special studies to assess pharmacological actions other than the intended therapeutic effect(s)).

(b) *Pharmacokinetics and Product Metabolism in Animals.* A summary of the pharmacokinetics and biological transformation and disposition of the investigational product in all species studied should be given. The discussion of the findings should address the absorption and the local and systemic bioavailability of the investigational product and its metabolites, and their relationship to the pharmacological and toxicological findings in animal species.

(c) *Toxicology.* A summary of the toxicological effects found in relevant studies conducted in different animal species should be described under the following headings where appropriate:

- Single dose
- Repeated dose
- Carcinogenicity
- Special studies (e.g., irritancy and sensitization)
- Reproductive toxicity
- Genotoxicity (mutagenicity)

6. *Effects in Humans.* A thorough discussion of the known effects of the investigational product(s) in humans should be provided, including information on pharmacokinetics, metabolism, pharmacodynamics, dose response, safety, efficacy, and other pharmacological activities. Where possible, a summary of each completed clinical trial should be provided. Information should also be provided regarding results of any use of the investigational product(s) other than from clinical trials, such as from experience during marketing.

(a) *Pharmacokinetics and Product Metabolism in Humans.* A summary of information on the pharmacokinetics of the investigational product(s) should be presented, including the following, if available:
  - Pharmacokinetics (including metabolism, as appropriate, and absorption, plasma protein binding, distribution, and elimination)
  - Bioavailability of the investigational product (absolute, where possible, and/or relative) using a reference dosage form
  - Population subgroups (e.g., gender, age, and impaired organ function)
  - Interactions (e.g., product–product interactions and effects of food)
  - Other pharmacokinetic data (e.g., results of population studies performed within clinical trial(s)

(b) *Safety and Efficacy.* A summary of information should be provided about the investigational product's/products' (including metabolites, where appropriate) safety, pharmacodynamics, efficacy, and dose response that were obtained from preceding trials in humans (healthy volunteers and/or patients). The implications of this information should be discussed. In cases where a number of clinical trials have been completed, the use of summaries of safety and efficacy across multiple trials by indications in subgroups may provide a clear presentation of the data. Tabular summaries of adverse drug reactions for all the clinical trials (including those for all the studied indications) would be useful. Important differences in adverse drug reaction patterns/incidences across indications or subgroups should be discussed.

   The IB should provide a description of the possible risks and adverse drug reactions to be anticipated on the basis of prior experiences with the product under investigation and with related products. A description should also be provided of the precautions or special monitoring to be done as part of the investigational use of the product(s).

(c) *Marketing Experience.* The IB should identify countries where the investigational product has been marketed or approved. Any significant information arising from the marketed use should be summarized (e.g., formulations, dosages, routes of administration, and adverse product reactions).

The IB should also identify all the countries where the investigational product did not receive approval/registration for marketing or was withdrawn from marketing/registration.

7. *Summary of Data and Guidance for the Investigator.* This section should provide an overall discussion of the nonclinical and clinical data, and should summarize the information from various sources on different aspects of the investigational product(s), wherever possible. In this way, the investigator can be provided with the most informative interpretation of the available data and with an assessment of the implications of the information for future clinical trials.

Where appropriate, the published reports on related products should be discussed. This could help the investigator to anticipate adverse drug reactions or other problems in clinical trials.

The overall aim of this section is to provide the investigator with a clear understanding of the possible risks and adverse reactions, and of the specific tests, observations, and precautions that may be needed for a clinical trial. This understanding should be based on the available physical, chemical, pharmaceutical, pharmacological, toxicological, and clinical information on the investigational product(s). Guidance should also be provided to the clinical investigator on the recognition and treatment of possible overdose and adverse drug reactions that are based on previous human experience and on the pharmacology of the investigational product.

CHAPTER 2

THERAPEUTIC PRODUCTS CLINICAL DEVELOPMENT IN THE UNITED STATES

2.1 DRUG DISCOVERY

Drug research is a complex, lengthy, and very costly process. Only 1 out of 5000 candidates may have the potential to reach the market. Although the pharmaceutical industry invests enormous resources to develop potential therapeutic agents, the time to completion and market application on average takes more than 8.5 years according to the FDA.

The drug development process starts with the **discovery** phase. During this period, hundreds of drug candidates are synthesized, modified, and evaluated for possible therapeutic applications according to the functional/therapeutic objectives sought after. In the case of biologicals, biomolecules are manufactured using different methods to obtain a viable biomolecule that can mimic a natural molecule or be enhanced structurally/functionally to affect a molecular process to treat a condition. Also, therapeutic agents can be products obtained from microorganisms such as fungi, viruses, and bacteria.

All these processes may yield candidates that will be either tested by computerized modeling and prediction techniques and/or further experimentally tested for possible preclinical development.

2.2 PRECLINICAL DEVELOPMENT

2.2.1 In Vitro Testing

Once the potential candidates have been identified, **preclinical** development is initiated. The products are tested initially **in vitro** for toxicology, genotoxicity, and biological activity. In vitro tests are not going to define in detail the toxicological profile of the product; however, they will provide an indication on the probability of which products may continue development for further human testing.

Clinical Trials Audit Preparation: A Guide for Good Clinical Practice (GCP) Inspections, by Vera Mihajlovic-Madzarevic
Copyright © 2010 John Wiley & Sons, Inc.

2.2.2   In Vivo Testing (Animal Testing)

To proceed with clinical development, the FDA requires that a sponsor submits data showing that the drug is reasonably safe for use in initial, small-scale clinical studies (submission of an Investigational Drug Application—IND).

Data may be gathered for an Investigational Drug Application using different approaches: (1) compiling existing nonclinical data from past **in vitro** laboratory or animal studies on the compound; (2) compiling data from previous clinical testing or marketing of the drug in the United States or another country whose population is relevant to the U.S. population; or (3) undertaking new preclinical studies designed to provide the evidence necessary to support the safety of administering the compound to humans.

During this period in development, the products that seem viable to test in animals (**in vivo testing**) are undertaken for the following reasons:

1. Develop a pharmacological profile of the drug.
   (a) Absorption, distribution, metabolism, and elimination (ADME).
   (b) Mode of action. (These studies are limited by the ability to gather information on endpoints at the molecular level relevant to human therapeutics— that is, limited to data that does not involve subject interview.)
2. Determine the acute toxicity of the drug in at least two species of animals.
3. Conduct short-term toxicity studies ranging from 2 weeks to 3 months or more, depending on the proposed duration of use of the substance in the proposed clinical studies.

Animal studies should be performed in at least two species of animals—one of them nonrodent. Also, these studies have to demonstrate a certain degree of safety and therapeutic potential to support an Investigational New Drug Application.

Note that long-term toxicity studies may continue during this stage of development well past the clinical stage. The animal data obtained from these studies are very important to support further clinical safety if the product is going to be used for long-term treatment in humans.

The animal studies in the preclinical phase must be conducted in strict adherence to Good Laboratory Practice.[1]

Parallel to preclinical development, the pharmaceutical sponsor has to develop a process to manufacture small-scale investigational product that will be used during the clinical phases. This parallel manufacturing development process has to comply with Good Manufacturing Practice (GMP) for investigational products.

2.3   CLINICAL DEVELOPMENT

To enter clinical development, a comprehensive risk assessment should be performed as to whether the investigational product is safe enough to expose human subjects.

---

[1] Title 21 Food and Drugs Chapter 1, Food and Drug Administration Department of Health and Human Services, Subchapter A, General, Part 58, Good Laboratory Practices for Non Clinical Laboratory Studies (Rev. April 1, 2008).

Therefore, once the pharmaceutical company developing a therapeutic product is able to demonstrate that the product has an acceptable safety profile in animals and potential therapeutic use in humans and the Investigational New Drug Application has been approved by the FDA, it is ready to start clinical development. Nevertheless, the FDA has tools to stop development at any point if it is not convinced that the data presented demonstrates an acceptable risk to patients, therefore issuing a **clinical hold**.

Clinical development is performed in human subjects (healthy volunteers and patients who have the condition for which the product is being developed). Clinical development to gather safety and efficacy data for market application is comprised by three main phases.

1. *Phase I*. In this phase the product is tested for the *first time in human volunteers* to determine the pharmacokinetic parameters of the drug and initial safety. Phase I studies are short and can employ single or multiple doses. Also, in these studies early evidence of efficacy is intended to be collected, if possible. (The exception is oncology drug development where Phases I and II can be conducted simultaneously in patients). In summary, Phase I studies:

   - Are conducted in healthy volunteers
   - Have a small number of subjects (20–80)
   - Are short-term studies
   - Examine pharmacokinetics and initial safety
   - Give early evidence of efficacy (if leads are identified)

2. *Phase II*. The drug is tested in patients in early controlled studies. The total number of patients exposed in this phase is on the order of hundreds. The patients selected must have the condition for which the drug is to be developed. These studies are to determine the initial safety and efficacy of the investigational product in a particular indication in patients, as well as tolerability and dose finding. This phase may last a couple of years until safety and efficacy is determined as well as optimal doses. In summary, Phase II studies:

   - Are conducted in patients
   - Have number of subjects in the range of 50 to hundreds per trial
   - Are longer-term studies (weeks to months)
   - Examine safety and tolerability
   - Determine initial efficacy and dose finding

3. *Phase III*. In this phase we do include *pivotal studies*. These studies are going to provide most of the safety and efficacy data initially gathered in Phase II in a smaller number of patients, for the market application (NDA—New Drug Application). These studies can be either controlled or uncontrolled. The total number of patients exposed in these studies will be on the order of thousands. The larger sample size will allow collecting adequate safety and efficacy

information to determine statistically significant differences between treatment groups. In summary, Phase III studies:

- Are conducted in patients
- Have hundreds to thousands of subjects per trial
- Are longer-term studies (weeks to months)
- Are pivotal studies
- Examine safety and efficacy
- Are comparative studies
- Are controlled and uncontrolled

2.4 FDA CONSIDERATIONS FOR DRUG DEVELOPMENT

The FDA encourages a fluent dialog between the sponsor and the agency during the drug development process and even before a drug enters clinical development. This will allow both parties to become familiar with the process and the investigational product. It is very important that the sponsor initiates this early communication as soon as it has initial preclinical data to avoid unnecessary studies or submit an IND with limited data and go back to square one.

2.4.1 Pre-IND Meeting

These meetings are initiated by the sponsor before or during animal testing. The team that is going to review the information presented will be the same one to further review the application. These meetings are useful to determine (1) testing phases, (2) data requirements, and (3) any scientific issues that may need to be resolved prior to IND submission. The sponsor and FDA discuss and agree upon the design of the animal studies needed to initiate human trials.

2.4.2 End of Phase II Meeting

This meeting is initiated by the sponsor. To prepare for the meeting, one month before the end of Phase II the sponsor must submit background information and the protocols for Phase III. This will provide the review team with information needed to prepare for a productive meeting. The information submitted prior to the meeting should be:

- Data supporting the claim of the new drug product
- Chemistry data
- Animal data
- Proposed additional animal data

- Results of Phase I and II studies
- Statistical methods being used
- Specific protocols for Phase III studies
- A copy of the proposed labeling for a drug, if available

The primary objective of the "end of Phase II" meetings is (1) to determine whether it is safe to begin Phase III testing, (2) to plan protocols for Phase III human studies, and (3) to discuss and identify any additional information that may be required to support the submission of a new drug application. It is also intended to establish an agreement between the FDA and the sponsor of the overall plan for Phase III and the objectives and design of particular studies, and to allow data clarification in a timely manner to avoid unnecessary delays and expenditures.

2.4.3 Pre-NDA Meeting

The objective of the pre-NDA meeting is to discuss the presentation of all safety and efficacy data (paper and electronic) in support of the marketing application. The information the sponsor has to provide for the pre-NDA meeting is (1) a summary of clinical studies to be submitted in the NDA; (2) the proposed format for organizing the submission, including methods for presenting the data; and (3) other information needed to be discussed.

The ultimate objective of the pre-NDA meeting is (1) to uncover any major unresolved problems or issues, (2) to identify studies the sponsor is relying on as adequate and well controlled in establishing the effectiveness of the drug, (3) to help the reviewers become familiar with the general information to be submitted, and (4) to discuss the presentation of the data in the NDA to facilitate its review.

If certain matters do not become obvious during this meeting, the FDA may request a meeting 90 days after the initial submission in order to clarify any outstanding issue.

2.5   PHASE IV, POSTMARKETING SURVEILLANCE AND GCP

Phase IV studies or postmarketing studies have been developed to gather postmarketing data on therapeutic products as a follow-up mainly on unexpected safety issues. Another objective is to demonstrate that efficacy in the real clinical setting is concurrent with the premarket experience.

It is important to note the difference between what a Phase IV study is and postmarketing surveillance. Phase IV studies are run according to a protocol and certain defined criteria and data is analyzed further. On the other hand, routine postmarketing surveillance is performed continuously from reports originated by practitioners and manufacturers to comply with safety reporting according to the FDA 21 CFR 53 "Postmarketing Surveillance and Epidemiology: Human Drugs."

Phase IV studies are carried out when a sponsor/manufacturer of a marketed product intends to further test in patients the specified product for the same indication and in the same dosage form as approved. Furthermore, if an approved product has to be tested in a new indication, the sponsor must file a new IND and go back to Phase III. Additionally, if the dosage form targeted is different from the approved form, the sponsor must perform bioequivalence studies to demonstrate identity or run new Phase I trials to obtain pharmacokinetic data of the new dosage form.

Although clinical trial data is critical for the marketing approval on a new therapeutic product, it has its limitations due to sample size studied and extent of exposure of the study subjects. Therefore, we may not have had the chance to observe certain adverse events that are either rare or due to long-term exposure.

Postmarketing studies are conducted in a less stringent manner because GCP compliance is not generally required in the United States. Nevertheless, the limited approach on data collection could not allow concluding far beyond the power of the method. Also, and due to recent safety issues linked to antidepressants and COX-2 inhibitors, there is a greater necessity to reevaluate the importance of postmarketing studies other than depending on surveillance programs.

Having clarified what Phase IV studies entitle, it is very important that sponsors proceed with further studies to be performed on marketed products to demonstrate safety and efficacy in the "real world" scenario, where the limitations of the pre-clinical settings are reduced and where a larger sample size can be achieved. With analysis of the results of these types of studies, the sponsor should either (1) be able to demonstrate concurrence with the safety and efficacy data gathered during clinical development, or (2) reassess safety and efficacy and indicate where the new information diverges from the original assumptions. Any divergence can seriously affect the labeling of the product and future marketability.

There is also a trend now from regulators such as the FDA to require Phase IV (commitments) studies of marketed products and to bind the results on future marketability and labeling of the approved product.

Unlike for Phase IV studies, the FDA has a clear inspectional strategy to determine whether drug applicants (drug manufacturers, packers, and own label distributors) submit all required postmarketing Adverse Drug Experiences (ADE) reports to the agency, and whether ADE reports are complete, accurate, and submitted in accordance with reporting time frames. Failure to submit on time or follow up on serious ADEs may severely impact the future marketability of the product.

2.6 QUALITY ASSURANCE IN CLINICAL RESEARCH

Good Clinical Practice establishes that sponsors and Institutional Review Boards (IRBs) should implement standard operating procedures (SOPs) to ensure that the activities carried out are in compliance with GCP and regulatory requirements. The investigator is not required as per GCP to implement SOPs to ensure compliance; however, it is a requirement to adhere to the protocol and the procedures described. Note that certain regulatory bodies, such as the Therapeutic Drug Directorate of Health Canada, do extend the requirement to investigators.

SOPs assist the sponsor and IRBs to interpret and incorporate those requirements and guidelines into their clinical research activities.

To ensure compliance the parties should (1) have SOPs, (2) train the personnel
implementing those procedures periodically, (3) update the procedures, and (4) have
an independent quality assurance unit with an internal inspectional policy to ensure
adherence to SOPs, GCP, and regulatory requirements. The latter is very important,
since regulatory inspectional observations may focus on the fact that stakeholders
having SOPs do not have QA systems in place to ensure adherence.

2.7   FDA INSPECTIONAL BACKGROUND AND DATA

2.7.1   The FDA and GCP

The FDA,[2] a party to the International Conference on Harmonization of Technical
Requirements for Registration of Pharmaceuticals for Human Use, agreed to be observant of GCP in April 1996 together with Japan and the European Union. The
guidance was published in the *Federal Register* on May 9, 1997 (62 FR 25692).
Also, the FDA implemented a Good Clinical Practice Program, where Good Clinical
Practice issues arising in human research trials regulated by the FDA are attended.
Among others, the Good Clinical Practice Program coordinates FDA policies, coordinates the FDA's Bioresearch Monitoring Program with respect to clinical trials,
working together with FDA's Office of Regulatory Affairs (ORA), and contributes to
international GCP harmonization activities. It is important to highlight that the FDA
requires that GCP guidelines be observed for Phases I–III of clinical development
while the EU Directives cover all phases of clinical research, including postmarketing
(Phase IV) trials.

Note that the FDA has regulations that directly relate to GCPs as follows:

- Electronic Records; Electronic Signatures (21 CFR Part 11)
- Protection of Human Subjects (Informed Consent) (21 CFR Part 50)
- Financial Disclosure by Clinical Investigators (21 CFR Part 54)
- Institutional Review Boards (21 CFR Part 56)
- Investigational New Drug Application (21 CFR Part 312)
- Foreign Clinical Trials Not Conducted Under an IND (21 CFR Part 312.120)
- Forms 1571 (Investigational New Drug Application) and 1572 (Statement of
  Investigator)
- Applications for FDA Approval to Market a New Drug (21 CFR Part 314)
- Bioavailability and Bioequivalence Requirements (21 CFR Part 320)
- Applications for FDA Approval of a Biologic License (21 CFR Part 601)
- Investigational Device Exemptions (21 CFR Part 812)
- Premarket Approval of Medical Devices (21 CFR Part 814)

[2]http://www.fda.gov/cder/audiences/iact/forum/200710_samuels.pdf.

These regulations became very relevant from the QA aspect since it is important to emphasize that the inspectional strategies are based on the stakeholder's comparison of practices and procedures against regulatory requirements (above) and GCP.

The following are the responsibilities that sponsors, investigators and institutional review boards assume in an FDA study.

2.7.2 FDA: Responsibilities of the Sponsor (Subpart D 21 CFR 312.50 to 21 CFR 312.58)

GCP is an international guideline and applies to all clinical trials; however, it specifically makes reference to each country's particular requirements that have to be observed as well as the applicability of GCP. The FDA takes a leading role in that aspect with requirements for sponsors as follows:

(a) Selecting qualified investigators,

(b) Providing them with the information they need to conduct an investigation properly,

(c) Ensuring proper monitoring of the investigation(s),

(d) Ensuring that the investigation(s) is conducted in accordance with the general investigational plan and protocols contained in the IND,

(e) Maintaining an effective IND with respect to the investigations, and

(f) Ensuring that FDA and all participating investigators are promptly informed of significant new adverse effects or risks with respect to the drug.

(g) A sponsor may transfer responsibility for any or all of the obligations set forth in this part to a contract research organization. Any such transfer shall be described in writing. If not all obligations are transferred, the writing is required to describe each of the obligations being assumed by the contract research organization.

The sponsor of a clinical trial is also responsible for selecting investigators and monitors as follows:

(a) *Selecting Investigators.* A sponsor shall select only investigators qualified by training and experience as appropriate experts to investigate the drug.

(b) *Control of Drug.* A sponsor shall ship investigational new drugs only to investigators participating in the investigation.

(c) *Obtaining Information from the Investigator.* Before permitting an investigator to begin participation in an investigation, the sponsor shall obtain the following:

(i) A signed investigator statement (Form FDA-1572) containing:

(i) The name and address of the investigator;

(ii) The name and code number, if any, of the protocol(s) in the IND identifying the study(ies) to be conducted by the investigator;

(iii) The name and address of any medical school, hospital, or other research facility where the clinical investigation(s) will be conducted;

(iv) The name and address of any clinical laboratory facilities to be used in the study;

(v) The name and address of the IRB that is responsible for review and approval of the study(ies);

(vi) A commitment by the investigator that he or she:

1. Will conduct the study(ies) in accordance with the relevant, current protocol(s) and will only make changes in a protocol after notifying the sponsor, except when necessary to protect the safety, the rights, or welfare of subjects;

2. Will comply with all requirements regarding the obligations of clinical investigators and all other pertinent requirements in this part;

3. Will personally conduct or supervise the described investigation(s);

4. Will inform any potential subjects that the drugs are being used for investigational purposes and will ensure that the requirements relating to obtaining informed consent (21 CFR part 50) and institutional review board review and approval (21 CFR part 56) are met;

5. Will report to the sponsor adverse experiences that occur in the course of the investigation(s) in accordance with 312.64;

6. Has read and understands the information in the investigator's brochure, including the potential risks and side effects of the drug; and

7. Will ensure that all associates, colleagues, and employees assisting in the conduct of the study(ies) are informed about their obligations in meeting the above commitments.

8. A commitment by the investigator that, for an investigation subject to an institutional review requirement under part 56, an IRB that complies with the requirements of that part will be responsible for the initial and continuing review and approval of the clinical investigation and that the investigator will promptly report to the IRB all changes in the research activity and all unanticipated problems involving risks to human subjects or others, and will not make any changes in the research without IRB approval, except where necessary to eliminate apparent immediate hazards to the human subjects.

9. A list of the names of the subinvestigators (e.g., research fellows, residents) who will be assisting the investigator in the conduct of the investigation(s).

(ii) *Curriculum Vitae.* A curriculum vitae or other statement of qualifications of the investigator showing the education, training, and experience that qualifies the investigator as an expert in the clinical investigation of the drug for the use under investigation.

(iii) *Clinical Protocol*

1. For Phase I investigations, a general outline of the planned investigation including the estimated duration of the study and the maximum number of subjects that will be involved.

2. For Phase II or III investigations, an outline of the study protocol including an approximation of the number of subjects to be treated with the drug and the number to be employed as controls, if any; the clinical uses to be investigated; characteristics of subjects by age, sex, and condition; the kind of clinical observations and laboratory tests to be conducted; the estimated duration of the study; and copies or a description of case report forms to be used.

(iv) *Financial Disclosure Information.* Sufficient accurate financial information to allow the sponsor to submit complete and accurate certification or disclosure statements required under part 54 of this chapter. The sponsor shall obtain a commitment from the clinical investigator to promptly update this information if any relevant changes occur during the course of the investigation and for 1 year following the completion of the study.

(v) *Selecting Monitors.* A sponsor shall select a monitor qualified by training and experience to monitor the progress of the investigation

(vi) In the case of emergency research the sponsor has additional responsibilities, as stated in 21 CRF 312 50.24.

2.7.3   FDA: Responsibilities of the Investigator – (Subpart D 21 CFR 312.50 to 21 CFR 312.58)

The general responsibilities of an investigator as well as requirements for an investigator are stated in the *Code of Federal Regulations.* Every investigator must know these responsibilities **before** signing a Form 1572.

An investigator is responsible for (1) ensuring that an investigation is conducted according to the signed investigator statement, the investigational plan (protocol), and applicable regulations; (2) protecting the rights, safety, and welfare of subjects under the investigator's care; and (3) control of drugs under investigation.

An investigator shall, in accordance with the provisions of part 50 of this chapter; (1) obtain the informed consent of each human subject to whom the drug is administered, (2) **except** as provided in Section 50.23 or 50.24 of this chapter.

Note that the code is specific that "*additional specific responsibilities of clinical investigators are set forth in this part and in parts 50 and 56 of this chapter.*"

An investigator is also responsible for the control of the investigational drug:

- An investigator shall administer the drug only to subjects under the investigator's personal supervision or under the supervision of a subinvestigator responsible to the investigator.

- The investigator shall not supply the investigational drug to any person not authorized under this part to receive it.

Investigator Recordkeeping and Record Retention

(a) *Disposition of Drug.* An investigator is required to maintain adequate records of the disposition of the drug, including dates, quantity, and use by subjects. If the investigation is terminated, suspended, discontinued, or completed, the investigator shall return the unused supplies of the drug to the sponsor, or otherwise provide for disposition of the unused supplies of the drug under § 312.59.

(b) *Case Histories.* An investigator is required to prepare and maintain adequate and accurate case histories that record all observations and other data pertinent to the investigation on each individual administered the investigational drug or employed as a control in the investigation. Case histories include the case report forms and supporting data including, for example, signed and dated consent forms and medical records including, for example, progress notes of the physician, the individual's hospital chart(s), and the nurses' notes. The case history for each individual shall document that informed consent was obtained prior to participation in the study.

(c) *Record Retention.* An investigator shall retain records required to be maintained under this part for a period of 2 years following the date a marketing application is approved for the drug for the indication for which it is being investigated; or, if no application is to be filed or if the application is not approved for such indication, until 2 years after the investigation is discontinued and FDA is notified.

Investigator Reports

(a) *Progress Reports.* The investigator shall furnish all reports to the sponsor of the drug who is responsible for collecting and evaluating the results obtained. The sponsor is required under 312.33 to submit annual reports to FDA on the progress of the clinical investigations.

(b) *Safety Reports.* An investigator shall promptly report to the sponsor any adverse effect that may reasonably be regarded as caused by, or probably caused by, the drug. If the adverse effect is alarming, the investigator shall report the adverse effect immediately.

(c) *Final Report.* An investigator shall provide the sponsor with an adequate report shortly after completion of the investigator's participation in the investigation.

(d) *Financial Disclosure Reports.* The clinical investigator shall provide the sponsor with sufficient accurate financial information to allow an applicant to submit complete and accurate certification or disclosure statements as required under part 54. The clinical investigator shall promptly update this information if any relevant changes occur during the course of the investigation and for 1 year following the completion of the study.

Assurance of IRB Review

An investigator shall assure that an IRB that complies with the requirements set forth in part 56 will be responsible for the initial and continuing review and approval of the proposed clinical study. The investigator shall also assure that he or she will promptly report to the IRB all changes in the research activity and all unanticipated problems involving risk to human subjects or others, and that he or she will not make any changes in the research without IRB approval, except where necessary to eliminate apparent immediate hazards to human subjects.

Inspection of Investigator's Records and Reports

An investigator shall upon request from any properly authorized officer or employee of the FDA, at reasonable times, permit such officer or employee to have access to, and copy and verify any records or reports made by the investigator pursuant to 312.62. The investigator is not required to divulge subject names unless the records of particular individuals require a more detailed study of the cases, or unless there is reason to believe that the records do not represent actual case studies, or do not represent actual results obtained.

Handling of Controlled Substances

If the investigational drug is subject to the Controlled Substances Act, the investigator shall take adequate precautions, including storage of the investigational drug in a securely locked, substantially constructed cabinet, or other securely locked, substantially constructed enclosure, access to which is limited, to prevent theft or diversion of the substance into illegal channels of distribution.

Disqualification of a Clinical Investigator

(a) If the FDA has information indicating that an investigator (including a sponsor–investigator) has repeatedly or deliberately failed to comply with the requirements of 21 CFR 312, part 50, or part 56, or has submitted to the FDA or to the sponsor false information in any required report, the Center for Drug Evaluation and Research or the Center for Biologics Evaluation and Research will furnish the investigator with a written notice of the matter complained of and offer the investigator an opportunity to explain the matter in writing, or, at the option of the investigator, in an informal conference. If an explanation is offered but not accepted by the Center for Drug Evaluation and Research or the Center for Biologics Evaluation and Research, the investigator will be given an opportunity for a regulatory hearing under part 16 on the question of whether the investigator is entitled to receive investigational new drugs.

(b) After evaluating all available information, including any explanation presented by the investigator, if the Commissioner determines that the investigator has repeatedly or deliberately failed to comply with the requirements of this part, part 50, or part 56, or has deliberately or repeatedly submitted false information to FDA or to the sponsor in any required report, the Commissioner will notify the investigator and the sponsor of any investigation in which the investigator has been named as a participant that the investigator is not entitled to receive investigational drugs. The notification will provide a statement of basis for such determination.

(c) Each IND and each approved application submitted under part 314 containing data reported by an investigator who has been determined to be ineligible to receive investigational drugs will be examined to determine whether the investigator has submitted unreliable data that are essential to the continuation of the investigation or essential to the approval of any marketing application.

(d) If the Commissioner determines, after the unreliable data submitted by the investigator are eliminated from consideration, that the data remaining are inadequate to support a conclusion that it is reasonably safe to continue the investigation, the Commissioner will notify the sponsor who shall have an opportunity for a regulatory hearing under part 16. If a danger to the public health exists, however, the Commissioner shall terminate the IND immediately and notify the sponsor of the determination. In such case, the sponsor shall have an opportunity for a regulatory hearing before FDA under part 16 on the question of whether the IND should be reinstated.

(e) If the Commissioner determines, after the unreliable data submitted by the investigator are eliminated from consideration, that the continued approval of the drug product for which the data were submitted cannot be justified, the Commissioner will proceed to withdraw approval of the drug product in accordance with the applicable provisions of the act.

(f) An investigator who has been determined to be ineligible to receive investigational drugs may be reinstated as eligible when the Commissioner determines that the investigator has presented adequate assurances that the investigator will employ investigational drugs solely in compliance with the provisions of this part and of parts 50 and 56.

2.7.4   FDA: Responsibilities of the Institutional Review Board – (21 CFR Part 56)

Circumstances in Which IRB Review is Required[3]

(a) Except as provided in 21 CFR 56.104 and 56.105, any clinical investigation which must meet the requirements for prior submission (as required in parts 312, 812, and 813) to the Food and Drug Administration shall not be initiated unless that investigation has been reviewed and approved by, and remains subject to continuing review by, an IRB meeting the requirements of this part.

(b) Except as provided in 21 CFR 56.104 and 56.105, the Food and Drug Administration may decide not to consider in support of an application for a research or marketing permit any data or information that has been derived from a clinical investigation that has not been approved by, and that was not subject to initial and continuing review by an IRB meeting the requirements of this part. The determination that a clinical investigation may not be considered in support of an application for a research or marketing permit does not, however, relieve the applicant for such a permit of any obligation under any other applicable regulations to submit the results of the investigation to the Food and Drug Administration.

(c) Compliance with these regulations will in no way render inapplicable pertinent Federal, State, or local laws or regulations.

Exemptions from IRB requirement

The following categories of clinical investigations are exempt from the requirements of this part for IRB review:

(a) Any investigation that commenced before July 27, 1981 and was subject to requirements for IRB review under FDA regulations before that date, provided that the investigation remains subject to review of an IRB which meets the FDA requirements in effect before July 27, 1981.

(b) Any investigation that commenced before July 27, 1981 and was not otherwise subject to requirements for IRB review under Food and Drug Administration regulations before that date.

(c) Emergency use of a test article, provided that such emergency use is reported to the IRB within 5 working days. Any subsequent use of the test article at the institution is subject to IRB review.

(d) Taste and food quality evaluations and consumer acceptance studies, if wholesome foods without additives are consumed or if a food is consumed that contains

---

[3] *Guidance for Industry: Using a Centralized IRB Review Process in Multicenter Clinical Trials.* U.S. Department of Health and Human Services, Food and Drug Administration Good Clinical Practice Program, Office of the Commissioner (OC), Center for Drug Evaluation and Research (CDER), Center for Biologics Evaluation and Research (CBER), Office of Regulatory Affairs (ORA), March 2006.

a food ingredient at or below the level and for a use found to be safe, or agricultural, chemical, or environmental contaminant at or below the level found to be safe, by the Food and Drug Administration or approved by the Environmental Protection Agency or the Food Safety and Inspection Service of the U.S. Department of Agriculture.

Waiver of IRB Requirement

On the application of a sponsor or sponsor–investigator, the Food and Drug Administration may waive any of the requirements contained in these regulations, including the requirements for IRB review, for specific research activities or for classes of research activities, otherwise covered by these regulations.

IRB Membership

(a) Each IRB shall have at least five members, with varying backgrounds to promote complete and adequate review of research activities commonly conducted by the institution. The IRB shall be sufficiently qualified through the experience and expertise of its members, and the diversity of the members, including consideration of race, gender, cultural backgrounds, and sensitivity to such issues as community attitudes, to promote respect for its advice and counsel in safeguarding the rights and welfare of human subjects. In addition to possessing the professional competence necessary to review the specific research activities, the IRB shall be able to ascertain the acceptability of proposed research in terms of institutional commitments and regulations, applicable law, and standards or professional conduct and practice. The IRB shall therefore include persons knowledgeable in these areas. If an IRB regularly reviews research that involves a vulnerable category of subjects, such as children, prisoners, pregnant women, or handicapped or mentally disabled persons, consideration shall be given to the inclusion of one or more individuals who are knowledgeable about and experienced in working with those subjects.

(b) Every nondiscriminatory effort will be made to ensure that no IRB consists entirely of men or entirely of women, including the institution's consideration of qualified persons of both sexes, so long as no selection is made to the IRB on the basis of gender. No IRB may consist entirely of members of one profession.

(c) Each IRB shall include at least one member whose primary concerns are in the scientific area and at least one member whose primary concerns are in nonscientific areas.

(d) Each IRB shall include at least one member who is not otherwise affiliated with the institution and who is not part of the immediate family of a person who is affiliated with the institution.

(e) No IRB may have a member participate in the IRB's initial or continuing review of any project in which the member has a conflicting interest, except to provide information requested by the IRB.

(f) An IRB may, at its discretion, invite individuals with competence in special areas to assist in the review of complex issues which require expertise beyond or in addition to that available on the IRB. These individuals may not vote with the IRB.

IRB Functions and Operations

In order to fulfill the requirements of these regulations, each IRB shall:

(a) Follow written procedures:

 (i) for conducting its initial and continuing review of research and for reporting its findings and actions to the investigator and the institution;

 (ii) for determining which projects require review more often than annually and which projects need verification from sources other than the investigator that no material changes have occurred since previous IRB review;

 (iii) for ensuring prompt reporting to the IRB of changes in research activity; and

 (iv) for ensuring that changes in approved research, during the period for which IRB approval has already been given, may not be initiated without IRB review and approval except where necessary to eliminate apparent immediate hazards to the human subjects.

(b) Follow written procedures for ensuring prompt reporting to the IRB, appropriate institutional officials, and the Food and Drug Administration of:

 (i) any unanticipated problems involving risks to human subjects or others;

 (ii) any instance of serious or continuing noncompliance with these regulations or the requirements or determinations of the IRB; or

 (iii) any suspension or termination of IRB approval.

(c) Except when an expedited review procedure is used (see 21 CFR 56.110), review proposed research at convened meetings at which a majority of the members of the IRB are present, including at least one member whose primary concerns are in nonscientific areas. In order for the research to be approved, it shall receive the approval of a majority of those members present at the meeting.

IRB Review of Research

(a) An IRB shall review and have authority to approve, require modifications in (to secure approval), or disapprove all research activities covered by these regulations.

(b) An IRB shall require that information given to subjects as part of informed consent is in accordance with 21 CFR 50.25. The IRB may require that information, in addition to that specifically mentioned in 21 CFR 50.25, be given to the subjects when in the IRB's judgment the information would meaningfully add to the protection of the rights and welfare of subjects.

(c) An IRB shall require documentation of informed consent in accordance with 21 CFR 50.27, except as follows:

 (1) The IRB may, for some or all subjects, waive the requirement that the subject, or the subject's legally authorized representative, sign a written consent form if it finds that the research presents no more than minimal risk of harm to subjects and involves no procedures for which written consent is normally required outside the research context; or

 (2) The IRB may, for some or all subjects, find that the requirements in 21 CFR 50.24 for an exception from informed consent for emergency research are met.

(d) In cases where the documentation requirement is waived as stated in 21 CFR 56 under paragraph (c)(1), where the IRB may require the investigator to provide subjects with a written statement regarding the research.

(e) An IRB shall notify investigators and the institution in writing of its decision to approve or disapprove the proposed research activity or of modifications required to secure IRB approval of the research activity. If the IRB decides to disapprove a research activity, it shall include in its written notification a statement of the reasons for its decision and give the investigator an opportunity to respond in person or in writing. For investigations involving an exception to informed consent under 50.24, an IRB shall promptly notify in writing the investigator and the sponsor of the research when an IRB determines that it cannot approve the research because it does not meet the criteria in the exception provided under 50.24(a) or because of other relevant ethical concerns. The written notification shall include a statement of the reasons for the IRB's determination.

(f) An IRB shall conduct continuing review of research covered by these regulations at intervals appropriate to the degree of risk, but not less than once per year, and shall have authority to observe or have a third party observe the consent process and the research. As of January 2010, there is a new draft guideline for continuing review of clinical research that may impact further the IRB responsibilities.[4]

(g) An IRB shall provide in writing to the sponsor of research involving an exception to informed consent under 21 CFR 50.24 a copy of information that has been publicly disclosed under paragraphs 50.24(a)(7)(ii) and (a)(7)(iii). The IRB shall provide this information to the sponsor promptly so that the sponsor is aware that such disclosure has occurred. Upon receipt, the sponsor shall provide copies of the information disclosed to FDA.

(h) When some or all of the subjects in a study are children, an IRB must determine that the research study is in compliance with 21 CFR part 50, subpart D, at the time of its initial review of the research. When some or all of the subjects in a study that is ongoing on April 30, 2001 are children, an IRB must conduct a review of the research to determine compliance with 21 CFR part 50, subpart D, either at the time of continuing review or, at the discretion of the IRB, at an earlier date.

Expedited Review Procedures for Certain Kinds of Research Involving No More than Minimal Risk and for Minor Changes in Approved Research

(a) The Food and Drug Administration has established, and published in the *Federal Register*, a list of categories of research that may be reviewed by the IRB through an expedited review procedure. The list will be amended, as appropriate, through periodic republication in the *Federal Register*.

(b) An IRB may use the expedited review procedure to review either or both of the following:

    1. some or all of the research appearing on the list and found by the reviewer(s) to involve no more than minimal risk,

---

[4]DRAFT-Guidance for IRBs, Clinical Investigators, and Sponsors. IRB Continuing Review after Clinical Investigation Approval, January 2010.

2. minor changes in previously approved research during the period (of 1 year or less) for which approval is authorized. Under an expedited review procedure, the review may be carried out by the IRB chairperson or by one or more experienced reviewers designated by the IRB chairperson from among the members of the IRB. In reviewing the research, the reviewers may exercise all of the authorities of the IRB except that the reviewers may not disapprove the research. A research activity may be disapproved only after review in accordance with the nonexpedited review procedure set forth in 56.108(c).

(c) Each IRB which uses an expedited review procedure shall adopt a method for keeping all members advised of research proposals which have been approved under the procedure.

(d) The Food and Drug Administration may restrict, suspend, or terminate an institution's or IRB's use of the expedited review procedure when necessary to protect the rights or welfare of subjects.

Criteria for IRB Approval of Research

In order to approve research covered by these regulations the IRB shall determine that all of the following requirements are satisfied:

1. Risks to subjects are minimized:

(i) by using procedures which are consistent with sound research design and which do not unnecessarily expose subjects to risk, and

(ii) whenever appropriate, by using procedures already being performed on the subjects for diagnostic or treatment purposes.

2. Risks to subjects are reasonable in relation to anticipated benefits, if any, to subjects, and the importance of the knowledge that may be expected to result. In evaluating risks and benefits, the IRB should consider only those risks and benefits that may result from the research (as distinguished from risks and benefits of therapies that subjects would receive even if not participating in the research). The IRB should not consider possible long-range effects of applying knowledge gained in the research (e.g., the possible effects of the research on public policy) as among those research risks that fall within the purview of its responsibility.

3. Selection of subjects is equitable. In making this assessment the IRB should take into account the purposes of the research and the setting in which the research will be conducted and should be particularly cognizant of the special problems of research involving vulnerable populations, such as children, prisoners, pregnant women, handicapped, or mentally disabled persons, or economically or educationally disadvantaged persons.

4. Informed consent will be sought from each prospective subject or the subject's legally authorized representative, in accordance with and to the extent required by 21 CFR part 50.

5. Informed consent will be appropriately documented, in accordance with and to the extent required by 21 CFR 50.27.

6. Where appropriate, the research plan makes adequate provision for monitoring the data collected to ensure the safety of subjects.

7. Where appropriate, there are adequate provisions to protect the privacy of subjects and to maintain the confidentiality of data.

8. When some or all of the subjects, such as children, prisoners, pregnant women, handicapped, or mentally disabled persons, or economically or educationally disadvantaged persons, are likely to be vulnerable to coercion or undue influence, additional safeguards have been included in the study to protect the rights and welfare of these subjects.

9. In order to approve research in which some or all of the subjects are children, an IRB must determine that all research is in compliance with 21 CFR part 50, subpart D.

Review by Institution

Research covered by these regulations that has been approved by an IRB may be subject to further appropriate review and approval or disapproval by officials of the institution. However, those officials may not approve the research if it has not been approved by an IRB.

Suspension or Termination of IRB Approval of Research

An IRB shall have authority to suspend or terminate approval of research that is not being conducted in accordance with the IRB's requirements or that has been associated with unexpected serious harm to subjects. Any suspension or termination of approval shall include a statement of the reasons for the IRB's action and shall be reported promptly to the investigator, appropriate institutional officials, and the Food and Drug Administration.

Cooperative Research

In complying with these regulations, institutions involved in multi-institutional studies may use joint review, reliance upon the review of another qualified IRB, or similar arrangements aimed at avoidance of duplication of effort.

IRB Records

(a) An institution, or where appropriate an IRB, shall prepare and maintain adequate documentation of IRB activities, including the following:

(1) Copies of all research proposals reviewed, scientific evaluations, if any, that accompany the proposals, approved sample consent documents, progress reports submitted by investigators, and reports of injuries to subjects.

(2) Minutes of IRB meetings which shall be in sufficient detail to show attendance at the meetings; actions taken by the IRB; the vote on these actions including the number of members voting for, against, and abstaining; the basis for requiring changes in or disapproving research; and a written summary of the discussion of controverted issues and their resolution.

(3) Records of continuing review activities.

(4) Copies of all correspondence between the IRB and the investigators.

(5) A list of IRB members identified by name; earned degrees; representative capacity; indications of experience such as board certifications, licenses, and so on, sufficient to describe each member's chief anticipated contributions to IRB deliberations; and any employment or other relationship between each member and the institution; for example, full-time employee, part-time

employee, a member of governing panel or board, stockholder, paid or unpaid consultant.

(6) Written procedures for the IRB as required by 21 CFR 56.108(a) and (b).

(7) Statements of significant new findings provided to subjects, as required by 21 CFR 50.25.

(b) The records required by this regulation shall be retained for at least 3 years after completion of the research, and the records shall be accessible for inspection and copying by authorized representatives of the Food and Drug Administration at reasonable times and in a reasonable manner.

(c) The Food and Drug Administration may refuse to consider a clinical investigation in support of an application for a research or marketing permit if the institution or the IRB that reviewed the investigation refuses to allow an inspection under this section.

Lesser Administrative Actions for Noncompliance

(a) If apparent noncompliance with these regulations in the operation of an IRB is observed by an FDA investigator during an inspection, the inspector will present an oral or written summary of observations to an appropriate representative of the IRB. The Food and Drug Administration may subsequently send a letter describing the noncompliance to the IRB and to the parent institution. The agency will require that the IRB or the parent institution respond to this letter within a time period specified by FDA and describe the corrective actions that will be taken by the IRB, the institution, or both to achieve compliance with these regulations.

(b) On the basis of the IRB's or the institution's response, FDA may schedule a reinspection to confirm the adequacy of corrective actions. In addition, until the IRB or the parent institution takes appropriate corrective action, the agency may:

1. Withhold approval of new studies subject to the requirements of this part that are conducted at the institution or reviewed by the IRB;

2. Direct that no new subjects be added to ongoing studies subject to this part;

3. Terminate ongoing studies subject to this part when doing so would not endanger the subjects; or

4. When the apparent noncompliance creates a significant threat to the rights and welfare of human subjects, notify relevant state and federal regulatory agencies and other parties with a direct interest in the agency's action of the deficiencies in the operation of the IRB.

(c) The parent institution is presumed to be responsible for the operation of an IRB, and the Food and Drug Administration will ordinarily direct any administrative action under this subpart against the institution. However, depending on the evidence of responsibility for deficiencies, determined during the investigation, the Food and Drug Administration may restrict its administrative actions to the IRB or to a component of the parent institution determined to be responsible for formal designation of the IRB.

Disqualification of an IRB or an Institution

(a) Whenever the IRB or the institution has failed to take adequate steps to correct the noncompliance stated in the letter sent by the agency under 56.120(a), and the Commissioner of Food and Drugs determines that this noncompliance may justify the disqualification of the IRB or of the parent institution, the Commissioner will institute proceedings in accordance with the requirements for a regulatory hearing set forth in part 16.

(b) The Commissioner may disqualify an IRB or the parent institution if the Commissioner determines that:

1. The IRB has refused or repeatedly failed to comply with any of the regulations set forth in this part, and

2. The noncompliance adversely affects the rights or welfare of the human subjects in a clinical investigation.

(c) If the Commissioner determines that disqualification is appropriate, the Commissioner will issue an order that explains the basis for the determination and that prescribes any actions to be taken with regard to ongoing clinical research conducted under the review of the IRB. The Food and Drug Administration will send notice of the disqualification to the IRB and the parent institution. Other parties with a direct interest, such as sponsors and clinical investigators, may also be sent a notice of the disqualification. In addition, the FDA may elect to publish a notice of its action in the *Federal Register*.

(d) The Food and Drug Administration will not approve an application for a research permit for a clinical investigation that is to be under the review of a disqualified IRB or that is to be conducted at a disqualified institution, and it may refuse to consider in support of a marketing permit the data from a clinical investigation that was reviewed by a disqualified IRB as conducted at a disqualified institution, unless the IRB or the parent institution is reinstated as provided in 56.123.

Public Disclosure of Information Regarding Revocation

A determination that the Food and Drug Administration has disqualified an institution and the administrative record regarding that determination are disclosable to the public under 21 CFR part 20.

Reinstatement of an IRB or an Institution

An IRB or an institution may be reinstated if the Commissioner determines, upon an evaluation of a written submission from the IRB or institution that explains the corrective action that the institution or IRB plans to take, that the IRB or institution has provided adequate assurance that it will operate in compliance with the standards set forth in this part. Notification of reinstatement shall be provided to all persons notified under 56.121(c).

Actions Alternative or Additional to Disqualification

Disqualification of an IRB or of an institution is independent of, and neither in lieu of nor a precondition to, other proceedings or actions authorized by the act. The Food and Drug Administration may, at any time, through the Department of Justice institute any appropriate judicial proceedings (civil or criminal) and any other appropriate regulatory action, in addition to or in lieu of, and before, at the time of, or after, disqualification. The FDA may also refer pertinent matters to another *Federal, State*, or local government agency for any action that that agency determines to be appropriate.

2.8   FDA BIORESEARCH MONITORING PROGRAM

2.8.1   Clinical Trials Inspectional Background

The FDA is one of the first regulatory agencies to conduct regular inspections of investigators, sponsors, and institutional review boards that are involved in clinical trials that intend to support a marketing application. The first disqualification of an investigator dates from 1964.

The FDA Bioresearch Monitoring program (BIMO) was initiated in 1977, incorporating the Clinical Inspection Program by the task force that included representatives for the areas of drugs, biologics, medical devices, and veterinary medicine and food. It was expanded to the CDRH (Center of Devices and Radiological Health) in June 1992. Under the Bioresearch Monitoring Program, the FDA conducts regulatory inspections of sponsors, institutional review boards, clinical investigators, and nonclinical laboratories involved in the testing of investigational products. Although ICH-GCP is not specifically defined in FDA regulations, one of the goals of BIMO is to demonstrate adherence to FDA-GCP.

2.8.2   Program Objectives

BIMO program consists primarily of on-site inspections and data audits designed to monitor all aspects of the conduct and reporting of FDA regulated research. The objectives of the inspection are described as follows:

- to assure the **quality and integrity of data** submitted to the FDA in support of new product approvals,
- to provide for **protection of the rights and welfare of human subjects** involved in FDA regulated research, and
- **to assure adherence** to FDA regulatory requirements and GCP.

    This program is the basis of the FDA preapproval process for new medicines, medical devices, food and color additives, and veterinary products introduced to the U.S. consumer.

2.8.3   Types of Inspections Performed by the FDA

BIMO inspections can be conducted at any stage of clinical development. The selection of sites to inspect will be done according to a set of criteria and program assignments. There are mainly two types of inspections: **routine** and **directed**.

Routine Inspections   These inspections are usually assigned after submission of an NDA, or marketing application of a therapeutic product. The routine assignments include inspections of clinical investigators, sponsors, IRBs, or nonclinical laboratories that are randomly selected for coverage under one of four compliance programs. These assignments are issued to monitor adherence to FDA regulations.

Directed (for Cause) Inspections These inspections are initiated when problems are identified during the FDA review process or due to complaints reported to the FDA from (1) other agencies, (2) sponsors or monitors, (3) institutions or institutional review boards, (4) site personnel, or (5) study subjects or the public.

Classification of Inspection Outcomes Classifications assigned to inspections indicate whether or not the establishment is operating in compliance with the regulations. The classification scheme used by the FDA is as follows:

- NAI—No Action Indicated: the inspected party is in compliance[5]
- VAI—Voluntary Action Indicated: minor deviations are observed, and voluntary correction action is requested from the inspected party[6]
- OAI—Official Action Indicated: serious noncompliance requiring regulatory or administrative action by the FDA against the inspected party (e.g., data unacceptable).[7]

2.8.4 Who Is Inspected?

- Clinical Investigator Sites
- Institutional Review Boards
- Sponsors, CRO's, Monitors of Clinical Investigations
- Bioequivalence Laboratories and Facilities
- Good Laboratory Practice (GLP) Inspections

2.8.5 Implementation of the FDA's Application Integrity Policy

The policy focuses on the integrity of data and information in applications submitted for Agency review and approval, formally entitled, "Fraud, Untrue Statements of Material Facts, Bribery, and Illegal Gratuities; Final Policy" (*Federal Register*, 56 FR 46191).

Implementation of the FDA's Application Integrity Policy involves investigations of sponsors that are suspected of submitting false or misleading data to the FDA. It also includes the review, evaluation, and monitoring of validity assessments required to be completed by sponsors found guilty of fraudulent activities.

---

[5]No Action Indicated (NAI). An NAI inspection classification occurs when no objectionable conditions or practices were found during the inspection or the significance of the documented objectionable conditions found does not justify further actions.

[6]Voluntary Action Indicated (VAI). A VAI inspection classification occurs when objectionable conditions or practices were found that do not meet the threshold of regulatory significance, but do warrant advisory actions to inform the establishment of findings that should be voluntarily corrected.

[7]Official Action Indicated (OAI). An OAI inspection classification occurs when significant objectionable conditions or practices were found and regulatory sanctions were warranted in order to address the establishment's lack of compliance with the regulation.

TABLE 2.1   FDA- BIMO Inspections for 2008

Center	Clinical investigators	IRBs	Sponsors/ monitors	GLP	Bioequivalence	Total
Center for Biologics Evaluation and Research (CBER)	77	19	6	4	NA	106
Center for Drug Evaluation and Research (CDER)	405	72	43	27	116	663
Center for Devices and Radiological Health (CDRH)	155	88	57	1	NA	301
Center for Food Safety and Applied Nutrition (CFSAN)	NA	NA	NA	1	NA	1
Center for Veterinary Medicine (CVM)	38	NA	3	14	NA	55

NA, not available.

2.8.6   BIMO Inspections for Clinical Trials

The Bioresearch Monitoring Program conducts inspections domestically and internationally. Every year the FDA conducts approximately 1100 GCP-BIMO inspections. The inspections are divided into four main groups: (1) clinical investigators, (2) institutional review board, (3) sponsors, CROs, and monitors, and (4) bioequivalence facilities/GLP inspections.

According to the FDA's HSP/BIMO Initiative Accomplishments update for 2008, a total of 1126 BIMO inspections were completed (see Table 2.1). Across all centers a total of 675 clinical investigator sites (excluding bioequivalence studies), 179 institutional review boards, 109 sponsors/CROs, and 47 GLP inspections were conducted.

A total of 705 clinical investigator sites were inspected (Figure 2.1). Of those, 50% were NAI (no action indicated) and therefore passed without regulatory observations; 41% were VAI (voluntary action indicated), where findings were

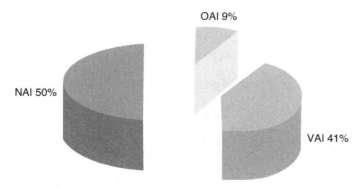

Figure 2.1   BIMO inspectional findings for clinical investigators (2008).

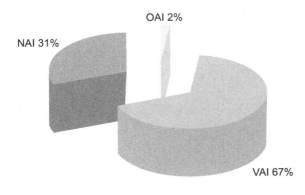

Figure 2.2 BIMO inspectional findings for bioequivalence studies (2008).

observed—however, they were not considered to be subject to mandatory action; and 9% were OAI (official action indicated), meaning that serious findings were observed and response was required before further action is started.

A total of 128 bioequivalence studies were inspected (Figure 2.2). Of those 31% were NAI (no action indicated) and therefore passed without regulatory observations; 67% were VAI (voluntary action indicated), where findings were observed—however, they were not considered to be subject to mandatory action; and 2% were OAI (official action indicated), meaning that serious findings were observed and response was required before further action is started.

A total of 90 sponsors/CROs were inspected (Figure 2.3). Of those, 61% were NAI (no action indicated) and therefore passed without regulatory observations; 20% were VAI (voluntary action indicated), where findings were observed—however, they were not considered to be subject to mandatory action; and 19% were OAI (official action indicated), meaning that serious findings were observed and response was required before further action is started.

A total of 188 institutional review boards were inspected (Figure 2.4). Of those, 46% were NAI (no action indicated) and therefore passed without regula-tory observations; 47% VAI were (voluntary action indicated), where findings were observed—however, they were not considered serious; and 7% were OAI (official action indicated), meaning that serious findings were observed and response was required before further action is started.

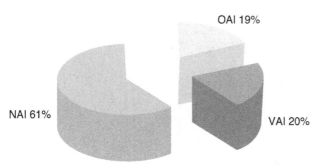

Figure 2.3 BIMO inspectional findings for sponsors/CRO (2008).

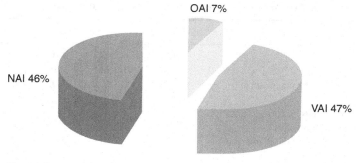

Figure 2.4   BIMO inspectional findings for IRB (2008).

According to the database Clinical Investigators Inspection List (CLIIL)[8] of the FDA for the year 2008, the data in Table 2.2 can be analyzed:

The table indicates that 54% of the BIMO-FDA inspections at clinical trial investigators sites are in compliance with regulatory requirements and GCP, and that about 92% are generally observant of the code of federal regulations.

Table 2.3 represents the number of findings to investigator site inspections where one site may have more than one finding. The finding for "All" represents the total number of findings since the database was built in 1977.

If we analyze the findings for the year 2008 according to the deficiency codes, we can represent them graphically as in Figure 2.5. Except for the code O0 (no deficiencies), we can observe that the code O5 (failure to follow investigational plan/protocol adherence) is represented in 29% (majority) of the observations in 2008 compared to 22% in All. Protocol adherence has been an issue since early inspections and was identified previously as the most observed finding in all inspections if we compare to the (All) data presented (see the comparative graph in Figure 2.6).

TABLE 2.2   BIMO Inspectional Findings for Clinical Investigators (2008)

Observation	Clinical sites	Percentage
NAI (no action indicated)	213	54.20
VAI1 (voluntary action indicated—correction made on site)	150	38.17
OAI (official action indicated)	5	1.27
VAI2 (voluntary action indicated—no response requested)	18	4.58
VAI3 (voluntary action indicated—response requested)	1	0.25
OAIC (official action indicated—completed)	1	0.25
OAIR (official action indicated—response requested)	1	0.25
OAIW (official action indicated—warning letter issued)	2	0.51
MTF (case closed with a memo to file)	2	0.51
Total	393	100

[8]http://www.accessdata.fda.gov/scripts/cder/cliil.

TABLE 2.3   Number of Findings According to the Deficiency Codes—2008 versus All

Codes[a]	2008	(%)	All	(%)
O0 (no deficiencies noted)	167	37.53	931	7.28
O1 (records availability)	4	0.90	189	1.48
O2 (failure to obtain and/or document subject consent)	16	3.60	247	1.93
O3 (inadequate informed consent form)	6	1.35	2552	19.95
O4 (inadequate drug accountability)	28	6.29	1328	10.38
O5 (failure to follow investigational plan)	131	29.44	2938	22.97
O6 (inadequate and inaccurate records)	69	15.51	2377	18.58
O7 (unapproved concomitant therapy)	3	0.67	190	1.49
O8 (inappropriate payment to volunteers)	0	0.00	24	0.19
O9 (unapproved use of drug before IND submission)	0	0.00	13	0.10
O1O (inappropriate delegation of authority)	0	0.00	59	0.46
O11 (inappropriate use/commercialization of IND)	0	0.00	15	0.12
O12 (failure to list additional investigators on form 1572)	0	0.00	107	0.84
O13 (subjects receiving simultaneous investigational drugs)	0	0.00	18	0.14
O14 (failure to obtain or document IRB approval)	0	0.00	193	1.51
O15 (failure to notify IRB of changes, failure to submit progress reports)	6	1.35	513	4.01
O16 (failure to report adverse drug reactions)	7	1.57	510	3.99
O17 (submission of false information)	0	0.00	78	0.61
O18 (other)	4	0.90	485	3.79
O19 (failure to supervise or personally conduct the clinical investigation)	4	0.90	15	0.12
O2O (failure to protect the rights, safety, and welfare of subjects)	0	0.00	10	0.08
O21 (failure to permit FDA access to records)	0	0.00	1	0.01
Total	445	100	12793	100

Codes 19, 20, and 21 became effective October 1, 2005.

A major observation was the code O6 (inadequate/inaccurate records), that is represented in 15% of the observations in 2008 compared to 18% in All.

However, we also can observe a new trend for the code O3 (inadequate informed consent form): whereas that code is represented in 19% of All observations, in 2008 that code is represented in only 1.3%. Another code related to the previous O2 (failure to obtain consent) in 2008 is represented 3.6% of cases compared to a total of 1.9% for All. This indicates that although there is a trend of improving in the consenting of subjects in clinical trials, there are still issues with *obtaining* the consent.

The other major finding is O4 (inadequate drug accountability) in 6% of the observations in 2008 compared to 10% for All, again showing a trend that drug accountability is being performed with more accuracy and in compliance.

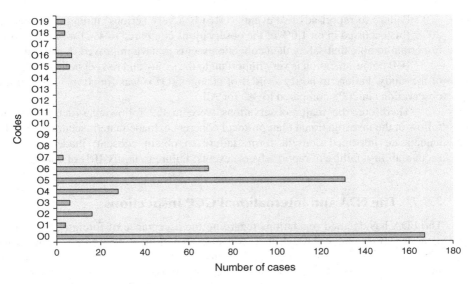

Figure 2.5 Deficiencies observed in 2008.

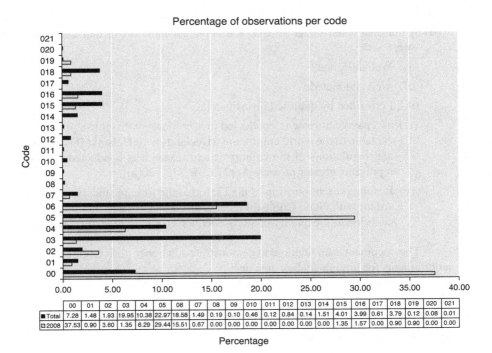

Figure 2.6 Comparative deficiencies observed in 2008 versus All.

Failure to report adverse events (O16) is a very serious finding; however, in 2008, this occurred in on 1.6% of the observations compared to 4% for All. It is very important to note that safety data collection seems to have improved in general.

IRB communication is very important to the safety and risk–benefit assessment of the study. Failure to notify an IRB of changes (O15) was found in 1.35% of the observations in 2008 compared to 4% for All.

Therefore, the major observations were in the following order: failure to follow in the investigational plan/protocol adherence; inadequate/inaccurate records; inadequate informed consent form; failure to obtain consent; inadequate drug accountability; failure to report adverse events; failure to notify IRB of changes.

2.8.7 The FDA and International GCP Inspections

The FDA has detailed regulations regarding the acceptance of foreign clinical trial data already available through their website. That clinical data may certainly contribute as non-U.S. data to FDA applications. The FDA sets conditions under which such data can be used in support of research or marketing in the United States.

Foreign studies should have been conducted in the following manner to support an application:

(**a**) If conducted under an IND, must comply with 21CRF312.

(**b**) If not conducted under an IND the applicant must prove that the study(ies) were:

(i) Well designed.

(ii) Well conducted.

(iii) Performed by qualified investigators.

(iv) as a past requirement: conducted in accordance with ethical principles acceptable to the world community (Declaration of Helsinki [DOH] or laws and regulations of the country where research is conducted, whichever represents greater protection) [21 CFR 312.120(a)].

(v) It is the present position of the FDA that the foreign studies must be consistent with Good Clinical Practice, providing broader and more detailed attention to the quality of study conduct as well as ethical principles.

The documentation required to demonstrate adherence and compliance to FDA requirements for foreign studies includes:

(i) Same items as 21 CFR 312.120 (b) (1) through (5), and

(ii) Names and qualifications of IEC (Independent Ethics Committees) members

(iii) Summary of IEC decision

(iv) Description of informed consent procedure

(v) Description of incentives, if any

(vi) Description of study monitoring

TABLE 2.4 Countries with Clinical Trial Sites Inspected by the FDA—Until 2007

Country	Number of inspections	Country	Number of inspections	Country	Number of inspections	Country	Number of inspections
Algeria[a]	1	Denmark	14	Italy	35	Poland	22
Argentina	16	Dominican Republic	1	Japan	3	Portugal	2
Australia	11	Egypt	1	Kenya	1	Romania	2
Austria	5	Estonia	4	Latvia	5	Russia	36
Bahamas	1	Finland	15	Lithuania	2	Slovenia	1
Belgium	26	France	54	Malawi	1	South Africa	30
Brazil	11	Gabon	1	Mexico	9	Spain	16
Canada	177	Germany	54	Netherlands	21	Sweden	31
Chile	5	Greece	2	New Zealand	3	Switzerland	1
China	6	Guatemala	2	Nigeria[a]	1	Taiwan	1
Colombia	1	Hong Kong	4	Norway	4	Thailand	4
Costa Rica	7	Hungary	9	Panama	2	United Kingdom	92
Croatia	3	Ireland	1	Peru	5	Venezuela	2
Czechoslovakia	13	Israel	4	Philippines	1	Zambia	1

[a]Data reviewed in United States.

Also, the FDA encourages sponsors of foreign trials to obtain written agreements with the investigators; however, that requirement may be waived upon request with justification.

In the case that the foreign data is the only support for a marketing application in the United State [21 CFR 314.106.(b)], the data should be:

(i) Applicable to the U.S. population and medical practice.

(ii) Studies are performed by investigators of recognized competence.

(iii) Data are considered valid without an on site inspection.

(iv) FDA is able to validate the data with an on site inspection.

Criteria for International Sites Selection for Inspection About 10% of the total clinical trials site inspections are of international sites and in the year 2007 the FDA conducted 134 foreign inspections. The FDA has criteria for inspections of foreign sites as follows: (1) if there is insufficient U.S. data, only foreign data is submitted to support an application, (2) domestic and foreign data show conflicting results important for decision making, or (3) there is a serious issue to resolve (e.g. suspicion of fraud, scientific misconduct, significant human protection violations).

To date, since the foreign inspectional strategy was implemented (1980–2007), Canada is the country with the most FDA inspections (177), followed by the United Kingdom (92) and France (54) (See Table 2.4.)

CHAPTER 3

THE INSPECTION PREPARATION

In this chapter the reader will be walked through the process of preparation for an inspection. GCP Inspections can be (1) **internal** to satisfy the sponsors' responsibility on implementation of a quality assurance program to ensure adherence to company standard operating procedures (SOPs), regulatory requirements, and Good Clinical Practice; or (2) **external**, that is, performed by a regulatory body to ensure data credibility, that the patients' rights and well-being are considered, and that specific regulatory requirements are followed. (See Table 3.1.)

It very important to understand that **"the best way to prepare for an audit or inspection is to implement processes and procedures to avoid noncompliant activities."**

3.1   CONDUCT OF AN INTERNAL GCP INSPECTION: QUALITY ASSURANCE INSPECTION

Commercial sponsors of clinical investigations, as in the case of the pharmaceutical industry, must have established quality assurance (QA) procedures for all regulated activities they perform as part of the quality policy of the company. Many companies follow standards such as ISO 9001 or other recognized quality management systems. It is important to underline that GCP inspections are recommended for all clinical trials conducted by sponsors including the periodical inspection of investigator sites as well as the sponsor's Trial Master Files to guarantee the quality of the data collected and adherence to requirements.

Noncommercial sponsors, as in the case of investigator-initiated studies, where investigators also assume the role of the sponsor, should also have quality assurance systems implemented to guarantee the quality of data and adherence to regulatory requirements. Often investigators who also assume the sponsor's responsibilities do not have a quality assurance system despite having SOPs and having assumed those responsibilities by signing FDA Form 1571--Investigational New Drug Application.

Institutional review boards are required to have SOPs and perform their duties according to GCP and regulatory requirements. Most IRBs fail to demonstrate that QA systems are in place to guarantee adherence to regulatory requirements.

The internal GCP quality assurance inspection can be (1) part of the regular QA program of the sponsor, or (2) as a result of an impending regulatory inspection

Clinical Trials Audit Preparation: A Guide for Good Clinical Practice (GCP) Inspections, by Vera Mihajlovic-Madzarevic
Copyright © 2010 John Wiley & Sons, Inc.

TABLE 3.1 GCP Inspections

Type	Who conducts the inspection	Purpose
Internal	Conducted by sponsor's QA team	Ensure adherence to company standard operating procedures, regulatory requirements, and Good Clinical Practice
External	Conducted by regulatory authorities	Ensure data credibility, that the patients' rights and well-being are considered and that specific regulatory requirements are followed

to an investigator site or within 6 months of submission of a New Drug Application (NDA). The conduct of the internal inspection should follow comparable practices and principles of the regulator and be as thorough as possible.

3.2 STEPS TO PREPARE FOR THE INTERNAL QA INSPECTION

3.2.1 Inspection of the Trial Master File (TMF)

The Trial Master File is an organized filing system that is located at the coordinating center of the clinical trial (the sponsor site or whoever assumes that responsibility) and contains all the essential documents for the conduct of a clinical study according to GCP and all regulatory documents (as required).

- The TMF should be set up according to the sponsor's procedures before a study starts.
- Access to the TMF should be restricted to authorized personnel only.
- Once documents are filed, retrieval should be avoided.
- Documents in the TMF may also be filed electronically, and in this case the systems should be set up to control access, printing, and copying privileges and be fully 21 CFR 11 compliant.
- It is recommended that the sponsor has a backup of all TMF documents in the case of loss or destruction. Specific procedures should be available in the company's procedures manual for that purpose.

The clinical research team of the sponsor should be aware of all internal SOPs, regulatory requirements and GCP, to complete the TMF in a dynamic manner.

There should also be an index of all filed documents with the description of the type of document and the date and place where it is filed in the TMF. Remember that easy access to documents is a must for a smooth running clinical trial. Access to documents will be scrutinized too.

3.2.2   Inspection of an Investigator Site

The monitor responsible for the site should advise the principal investigator during the Site Initiation Visit of the possibility of an inspection (internal or regulatory) to ensure during monitoring visits that the site is compliant and that the essential documents for clinical trials described in GCP and required by the regulator are always available.

On the other hand, the QA unit should have procedures to notify a site of an inspection visit. The monitor responsible for monitoring the site should also be notified. All inspection visits to a site should be scheduled to allow the site to prepare in advance all documents that are necessary for the inspection. The site should also be informed of the purpose and scope of the inspection and the outcome. It is expected that the investigator site will have the coordinator of the clinical study and the investigator available during the inspection. At the end of the inspection there should be a debriefing of the findings.

When serious violations are found, it is important to have a complete analysis of the impact of those findings. In some cases, and due to the nature of the noncompliance, the sponsor will not be able to utilize those data for the marketing submission and therefore the FDA should be notified (e.g., serious violations may imply that certain data were fabricated or that samples from patients were not obtained but are from another source). If the violations are of such a serious nature that falsification of data is suspected, the sponsor should investigate further to gather sufficient evidence, after which the sponsor should communicate to the FDA and exclude the data of that site from the analysis.

3.2.3   Inspection of the Contract Research Organization (CRO)

CROs are recognized by GCP and the regulations as service providers to the sponsors and, through a detailed written contract agreement, they assume certain sponsor responsibilities and therefore are accountable for their activities. The sponsor's QA unit should be able to periodically inspect CROs just as the regulator may do, to establish compliance and document all findings to be discussed to ensure corrective measures are set into place. It is important to note that the **sponsor retains all sponsor responsibilities at all times** regardless of contracting a CRO to perform activities on the sponsor's behalf, and therefore might be held accountable for third party violations. Also, the data gathered may not be eligible for marketing submission.

3.2.4   Inspection of Clinical Laboratories

This is the only point where clinical laboratories are discussed in this book. Clinical laboratory testing plays a very important role in the determination of safety parameters in clinical trials. The clinical lab results will provide most of the safety information for the study and efficacy, if appropriate. The quality assurance unit should also inspect the clinical laboratory before a study starts and thereafter periodically to establish adherence to GCP, GLP, the protocol, and other applicable requirements, and to determine that the tests have been performed in all subjects as agreed to and also, if data is transmitted electronically, compliance to all electronic data regulatory requirements. It is suggested that each and every laboratory is inspected to allow the sponsor to have more certainty on the quality of the safety data collected.

3.3 THE GCP QUALITY ASSURANCE UNIT

The company **quality assurance inspector(s) should be completely independent from the clinical activities** and that should be demonstrated in the company SOPs. The quality inspector should be qualified by background and experience to conduct internal GCP inspections and be continuously trained in the company SOPs, GCPs, and regulatory requirements. The sponsor must demonstrate that a quality unit and procedures exist together with an inspectional program; however, from the GCP point of view, it is not a requirement to have full-time GCP inspectors in house since the inspections are not mandatory after each and every study is completed and for each site. Therefore, depending on the sponsor's procedures, those inspections should be conducted periodically by an internal or a third party GCP inspector (contractor) to satisfy the requirement of QA and ensure compliance.

3.3.1 Scope of an Internal GCP Inspection

The internal QA inspection can occur **at any time** during the clinical trial. They could be **partial**—only one site or part of the TMF—or **complete**—where entire sites and the sponsor's data are audited. The scope of the internal inspection should be detailed in order to establish compliance to SOPs, regulatory requirements, and GCP.

Internally, the sponsor should have SOPs that will guide the clinical and QA personnel on the inspection procedures, as, for instance:

1. Notification of an impending internal inspection due to:
   (a) Sponsor's standard inspectional program for investigator sites and the TMF.
   (b) Inspection of a site that is monitored by a third party.
   (c) Inspection of a site due to problems detected by the monitor.
   (d) Preregulatory inspection of a site.
2. Role of the monitor of a site during an inspection. Those procedures may contain answers to the following topics:
   (a) Should the monitor visit the site before the internal auditor to prepare for the inspection?
   (b) Should the monitor of the site/project manager be available during the inspection?
3. Letter of inspection and inspection reports, and debriefing procedures.
4. Follow-up on internal inspectional findings, procedures, and responsibilities.

3.3.2   Outcome of an Internal Inspection

The QA inspector should discuss all findings with the principal investigator at the site or with the clinical team before leaving the premises as the regulatory inspector may do as well (see Table 3.2).

1. The QA inspector should issue an inspection certificate or **letter of inspection** to the investigator site or the party inspected stating the dates of inspection, the scope, and the name of the inspectors who visited the site. A copy of that letter should be filed in the TMF under QA of the study.

2. The QA inspector should also write a complete **inspection report** containing all findings regarding the company SOPs, regulatory requirements, and GCP. The **inspection report** is a confidential internal QA document that **is not filed in the TMF.**

3. The report should be presented to the party responsible for the clinical and regulatory team. A debriefing should be conducted on the findings, and **action should be taken immediately to correct any violations and deviations**.

4. If an investigator site was inspected, the site should also be **informed in writing** of the deviations and violations and together with the sponsor the site should implement remedial action to avoid noncompliant activities in the future.

5. It is of extreme importance to **document all these activities** since the FDA inspector may request access to internal inspection reports if deemed necessary as follows:

   (a) A letter of inspection is available in the files, but major violations have been observed. In that case the regulatory inspector may suspect (i) the appropriateness of the QA program and implementation, or (ii) that no action was taken on observations made after an internal inspection; therefore, a weak follow-up of inspectional observations may again target the QA program.

The request to the internal inspection report is done according to the **Compliance Policy Guide Sec. 130.300 "FDA Access to Results of Quality Assurance Program Audits and Inspections" (CPG 7151.02)** where the FDA announced its policy **not to review or copy a firm's records and reports that result from audits** of a quality assurance program when such audits are conducted according to a firm's written quality assurance program at any regulated entity. The intent of the policy is to encourage firms to conduct quality assurance program audits and inspections that are truthful and significant. According to FDA policy, The FDA will continue to review and copy records and reports of such audits and inspections in the following cases:

1. In "directed" or "for-cause" inspections and investigations of a sponsor or monitor of a clinical investigation.

2. In litigation (e.g., and not limited to, grand jury subpoenas, discovery, or other agency or Department of Justice law enforcement activity, including administrative regulatory actions).

3. During inspections made by inspection warrant, where access to records is authorized by statute.

4. When executing any judicial search warrant.

The Sponsor does not have any authority to inspect institutional review boards; however, it must demonstrate that the IRB reviewing the clinical trial is fully compliant to 21 CFR 56.

3.4 STEPS TO PREPARE FOR THE REGULATORY INSPECTION

The pharmaceutical, biotech, and medical devices industries are highly regulated and most of the activities are going to be inspected periodically to allow the continuance of their business.

A regulatory inspection is certainly a very stressful event, during which the inspected party is going to be scrutinized, exposed, and even sanctioned for failing to adhere to regulatory requirements. Although most of the companies and clinical investigators are aware of what is expected from them, findings are still common.

Investigator sites, IRBs, and sponsors may be **inspected at any time** during the course of the development of an investigational product.

Note that the **FDA-BIMO program** will conduct inspections of clinical trial sites, IRBs, and sponsors that perform clinical investigations on **FDA-regulated products**. And understand that the **FDA-BIMO program** inspectors will visit clinical trial sites, IRBs, and sponsors that perform clinical investigations of **FDA-regulated products** on human subjects regardless of the intention of the sponsor to apply for a marketing application.

What is an FDA regulated product? Basically, drugs or any other therapeutic agent (biologic or device) that is used or intended to be used to diagnose, treat, mitigate, or prevent a disease.

You, as the the prospective sponsor–investigator, should always submit an IND application if you plan to conduct clinical research on human subjects regardless of your intention to apply for a marketing application in the future (exceptions are exploratory research and medical practice).

Why submit an IND application? Human subjects have the same rights, as detailed in the Declaration of Helsinki, regardless of whether they participate in a clinical trial intended to support a market application or not. Remember that the "FDA is responsible for protecting the public health by assuring the safety, efficacy, and security of human and veterinary drugs, biological products, medical devices, our nation's food supply, cosmetics, and products that emit radiation."

TABLE 3.2 Internal GCP Quality Inspections

Party inspected	Conducted by	Notification	Place where inspection is conducted	Outcome	Follow-up
Sponsor	Sponsor's QA inspector	Clinical research team for the study and director	Sponsor TMF site; the same as in FDA Form 1571 IND application	Letter of inspection (filed in TMF) and inspection report (confidential, issued to clinical team director and QA unit)	Documentation on remedial actions taken and implemented (in the TMF); reinspection if necessary
Principal investigators	Sponsor's QA inspector	The principal investigator and the monitor for the study and management	At the investigator site (same address as indicated in FDA Form 1572)	Letter of inspection (filed in TMF) and inspection report (confidential, issued to clinical team director and QA unit), and letter to the investigator to explain the findings and to request implementation of remedial actions	Documentation on remedial actions taken and implemented (in the TMF); reinspection if necessary
CRO	Sponsor's QA inspector	CRO project responsible party—sponsor's study project manager	The same as in FDA Form 1571 IND application	Letter of inspection (filed in TMF) and inspection report, (confidential, issued to clinical team director, QA unit, and CRO project responsible party;) letter to the CRO requesting implementation of remedial actions	Follow-up with documentation on remedial actions taken and implemented; reinspection if necessary

TABLE 3.3 Clinical Investigator Inspection: The FDA Inspector's Call

Modality	Announced visit (phone call or letter)
Time frames	Within 10 working days of announcement
Tip	Do not request a delay for the inspection

3.5 CLINICAL INVESTIGATOR INSPECTIONS PREPARATION

Usually, FDA inspections of clinical investigators are **announced visits**. It is not the intention of the FDA inspector to make unannounced visits to the investigator site since availability of the principal investigators or personnel may be limited due to their other activities, mainly attending to patients. Nevertheless, the type of inspection may vary depending on the objective of the site visit. Therefore, the FDA conducts both announced and unannounced inspections of clinical investigator sites (1) to routinely verify data that has been submitted to the FDA; (2) as a result of a complaint to the FDA about the conduct of the study at the site; (3) in response to sponsor concerns or termination of the clinical site; (4) at the request of an FDA review division; and (5) related to certain classes of investigational products that the FDA has identified as products of special interest in its current work plan (i.e., targeted inspections based on current public health issues).

The inspector will announce his/her visit by telephone to the numbers provided in Form 1572. The time between the announcement of the visit and the actual visit is very short, sometimes 2 days but on average 10 days. It is recommended that investigators do not request a delay on the inspection date since it may not be positively regarded. (See Table 3.3).

Exceptions to the announcement of inspections at the investigator site are the "for-cause" investigations, where the inspection may be triggered by a serious complaint.

3.6 WHAT TO DO WHEN AN INVESTIGATOR SITE FDA INSPECTION IS ANNOUNCED

TIP: Do Not Panic! The clinical investigator should always be prepared to receive the inspector at any time.

When inspections are announced as part of a premarketing inspection strategy following an NDA submission, the clinical investigator should take the following actions:

1. If the study was sponsored by the industry, contact the sponsor immediately. The sponsor is not necessarily notified of a site inspection. The sponsor could also initiate the following activities to assist the site in the inspection:

   (a) Inform the CEO, president, vice president, all directors, and personnel involved with the clinical trial to be audited.

   (b) Plan and prepare a strategy for the inspection to assist the site.

(c) Organize a preregulatory audit/inspection.

(d) Conduct the internal audit ASAP and apply all remedial procedures immediately (contract a CRO if no personnel are available).

(e) Assess all possibilities and plan for possible regulatory findings.

(f) Provide regulatory and compliance support.

2. If it is an investigator-initiated study, the investigator should perform a preregulatory inspection to confirm the adherence to SOPs, GCP, and regulatory requirements.

3. Communicate the inspection to the institution (IRBs). Note that the FDA may, for efficiency, initiate a concurrent inspection for a previously uninspected IRB or an IRB that has not been inspected within the past 5 years.

Once the inspection has been communicated to the interested parties, the site has to prepare for the inspection in the following manner:

(a) According to the scope of the inspection that was explained to the investigator during the announcement of the inspection, the site must prepare all pertinent documentation. The documentation may comprise but is not all inclusive of that described in Table 3.4.

Remember to provide ONLY the documentation requested for the study to be audited; do NOT volunteer any additional irrelevant documents.

(b) The investigator site should prepare the place where the inspection will take place. Remember that inspectors are also people who work intensively, reading

TABLE 3.4   Documentation for an Inspection of an Investigator Site

The protocol and all amendments to the protocol	Form 1572
Source documents for all patients enrolled and patient files	The patient information and consent forms signed by the patients
All IRB documentation including the approved documents (protocol, consent forms, media ads)	The case report forms
The Investigator's Brochure and updates	SOPs if available
Documentation of delegation of responsibilities	Investigational product accountability logs
An organizational chart	The investigational product (if available)
Qualifications of personnel	Monitoring visit log
Electronic records and signatures procedures if relevant	All SAE reports with supporting data
Records retention procedures	Sponsor's correspondence
Laboratory normal values and laboratory certifications if local laboratory is used	Any other document that supports the clinical trial data
If it is a device study, all the provisions of 21 CFR 812	Audit certificates, if available

all the materials presented, and need a proper environment to be able to perform their duties.

   (i) The most appropriate is to have a meeting room within the facility or a clean empty office.

   (ii) If they are shared facilities, the investigator must make sure that the space is booked for a period of time.

   (iii) The inspector should also be provided with access to a phone and copying services.

   (iv) Places to avoid are master filing rooms, basements, and the doctor's office during patient visiting hours, as well as hallways, stairwells, and the cafeteria.

(c) The investigator as well as the coordinator must be available during the inspection.

(d) The investigator site must ensure that there is a responsible person who will photocopy all materials requested by the inspectors **personally**. At that time, a **second copy** must be generated should an observation arise for the investigator. In that case, the investigator will have replicated all documentation that the inspector collected as evidence for future reference. The investigator must make sure that the originals remain at the site.

(e) If a pharmacist of the institution's pharmacy was responsible for the investigational product, the pharmacist should be notified, and he/she should also be available for the inspection, since the inspector will pay a visit to the pharmacy and check all investigational product accountability records for ongoing studies.

(f) If the investigational product is still available because is an ongoing study, the inspector may request to see it. Make sure that it is accounted for and organized according to the protocol criteria.

3.7 SPONSOR'S INSPECTION PREPARATION

First, we have to define who the sponsor is in the eyes of the regulator. The FDA defines a sponsor as a group that consists of those individuals, organizations, or corporations that initiate clinical investigations and have been so identified by the FDA through receipt of an investigational exemption, an Investigational New Drug application, or application for research or marketing permit for an article (IDE, PMA, IND, NDA). A sponsor is defined in regulations 21 CFR 312.3, 510.3(k), and 812.3(n). The monitors are those individuals who were selected by either a sponsor or CRO to oversee the clinical investigation (they may be an employee of the sponsor or CRO, or an independent consultant). All the activities of the monitor will be audited for compliance purposes.

Parties providing services to sponsors are also inspected. This group consists of those organizations or corporations which have entered into a contractual agreement with a sponsor to perform one or more of the obligations of a sponsor (e.g., design of protocol, selection of investigators and study monitors, evaluation of reports, and preparation of materials to be submitted to the FDA). In accord with 21 CFR 312.52 and 511.1(f), responsibility as well as authority may be transferred and thus the CRO becomes a regulated entity.

Note that the medical device regulations (21 CFR 812) do not contain provisions for CROs.

Inspections of sponsors of clinical investigators **are NOT announced visits** unless otherwise instructed by the assigning center. Therefore, a sponsor of clinical studies that involve FDA-regulated products may occur at any time of development. The rationale is that the majority of sponsors are companies that have a physical address as indicated on Form 1571 and personnel who can attend to an inspector at any time.

In most of the cases, the inspections are conducted as part of the premarketing approval program; therefore, a sponsor may expect an inspection at any time upon submission of a marketing application.

The sponsor must ensure that all documentation in the TMF is inspected by the QA unit periodically.

Clinical trial data can be inspected at any time during development; therefore, the sponsor should also be prepared to have regulatory inspectors pay visits at any time.

The sponsor should have written procedures within their quality assurance program to cover GCP inspections of data from clinical trials. All clinical and QA personnel have to be fully trained on these procedures. Documentation should be available at all times in the Trial Master Files to support all data submitted to the FDA. Access to the documents in the TMF should be limited to the clinical team to collect all documents requested by the inspector, including all SOPs pertinent to clinical research effective during the period inspected.

Do not provide unrestricted access to the Trial Master File: always have a person with access privileges assigned to collect and provide documentation requested.

Quality assurance personnel may also be involved in providing for archival history of SOPs and inspection reports if required.

3.8 WHAT TO DO WHEN SPONSORS FDA INSPECTOR ARRIVE UNANNOUNCED

Tip: Do Not Panic! The sponsor should always be prepared to receive the inspector at any time.

When inspections are part of a premarketing inspection strategy following an NDA submission the sponsor should take the following actions:

1. Immediately inform the CEO or president, vice president, all directors, and personnel involved with the clinical trial/NDA data to be audited.

TABLE 3.5   Documentation for an Inspection of a Sponsor of a Clinical Investigation: General

Relevant organizational charts that document structure and responsibilities for all activities involving investigational products

List of studies not included in the NDA/PMA with reason

List of all studies that are part of the NDA/PMA

All relevant SOPs effective at the time the clinical trials were on-going

Specific trial documents described in Table 3.6

The outcome of a failed audit may cost the company in share value and marketability of their products. The company may not be regarded as a compliant facility and therefore can lose credibility.

2. According to the scope of the inspection, which is explained by the auditor during the announcement of the inspection upon presentation of Form 482, the sponsor must prepare all pertinent documentation. The documentation may comprise but is not all inclusive of that described in Table 3.5.

3. The sponsor should provide for an appropriate place where the inspectors can review the documentation, usually an empty office or a meeting room with access to a phone and copying services.

4. Prepare all personnel for the inspection as part of the quality assurance training.

5. Assign a clinical or QA person to the inspectors to provide assistance at all times. That person will photocopy all materials requested by the inspectors **personally**. At that time, a **second copy** must be generated should an observation arise for the sponsor. Check also that all originals are replaced in the TMF.

6. Places to avoid for the FDA inspection are the Trial Master Filing room and an occupied office of the clinical team.

3.9   THE INSTITUTIONAL REVIEW BOARD INSPECTIONS PREPARATION

The FDA conducts IRB inspections to determine if IRBs are operating in compliance with current FDA regulations and statutory requirements and if the IRBs are following their own written procedures. The FDA regulations pertinent to IRBs include 21 CFR Part 50 (Protection of Human Subjects), Part 56 (Institutional Review Boards), Part 312 (Investigational New Drug Application), and Part 812 (Investigational Device Exemptions).

Note that having a clinical study approved by an IRB does not guarantee to the investigators and the sponsor that the ethical considerations of a study has been reviewed, assessed, and approved. A noncompliant IRB's approval is equivalent to the investigators and sponsor as not having approval at all.

TABLE 3.6 Documentation for the Sponsor's Inspection of a Particular Clinical Trial Data[a]

The protocol and all amendments to the protocol	List of all investigators
List of all IRBs including the ones that did not approve the study	List of outside services and contractors (CROs, laboratories, IRBs)
Copies of IRB approvals for the sites or investigators letter assuring IRB approval was obtained in writing	Copy of any written agreement transferring responsibilities
Site placement, initiation, and monitoring reports	Internal QA inspection certificates or letters (no reports)
	List of internally audited studies
Certificate of analysis of all investigational products and batches/lots shipped to the investigator	Investigational product return logs and/or disposition logs
Data verification forms (resolution of issues)	The patient information and consent forms and templates approved by IRBs
The case report forms completed and any supporting documents sent by the investigator	All SAE reports and supporting documents (narratives)
Documents to demonstrate investigator's product storage conditions and conditions during shipping to investigator site	Correspondence to investigators relating to SAEs
The Investigator's Brochure and updates	Labels of test articles
List of all monitors (for the studies being inspected) along with their job descriptions and qualifications	Investigational product accountability logs
All Form 1572—investigators agreements	The investigational product (if available—may be requested for sampling)
Electronic records and signatures procedures if relevant	Any other document that supports the clinical trial data
Records retention procedures	Other correspondence
If it is a device study, all the provisions of 21 CFR 812	Clinical trial reports, if available

[a]Financial agreements and records are not normally part of an inspection; however, they may be requested if deemed necessary.

All IRBs that intend to review and approve clinical trials **MUST be compliant to FDA requirements,** knowledgeable of all regulatory requirements for clinical trials and GCP, and develop and implement **SOPs** and **quality processes** to guarantee compliance.

The FDA developed a checklist to assist IRBs/institutions in evaluating procedures for the protection of human subjects of research. That checklist is titled "A Self-Evaluation Checklist for IRBs"[1]. The FDA considers that successful IRBs make use of written procedures that, in one way or another, cover a common core of topics. The checklist is presented as to what procedures the IRBs should have mostly written. Written procedures for some of the items are not specifically required by FDA regulations (e.g., policy regarding place and time of meeting) but are appropriate to consider when comprehensive procedures are being developed. All inspected IRBs are supposed to have all SOPs required in the list.

3.9.1 Central IRBs

Although local IRBs are the most common setting for ethics review, in multicenter trials we can have the scenario where the sponsor used a central IRB in order to streamline the approval process and avoid delays in duplication. Essentially all IRBs, institutional, local, central, or private, must demonstrate adherence to 21 CFR Part 50 (Protection of Human Subjects), Part 56 (Institutional Review Boards), and Part 312 (Investigational New Drug Application). Also, if the IRB functions are centralized, the review process should be consistent with the requirements of existing IRB regulations Section 56.114 (21 CFR 56.114, Cooperative Research), providing that "institutions involved in multi-institutional studies may use joint review, reliance upon the review of another qualified IRB, or similar arrangements aimed at avoidance of duplication of effort." A centralized IRB review process involves an agreement under which multiple study sites in a multicenter trial rely in whole or in part on the review of an IRB **other** than the IRB affiliated with the research site.

For multicenter studies, the **central IRB** is the IRB that conducts reviews on behalf of all study sites that agree to participate in the centralized review process. That agreement should be in writing. For sites at institutions that have an IRB that would ordinarily review research conducted at the site, the central IRB should reach agreement with the individual institutions participating in centralized review and those institutions' IRBs about how to apportion the review responsibilities between local IRBs and the central IRB (21 CFR 56.114) in writing.

The IRB's inspectional strategy involves two types of inspections:

1. *Surveillance.* These inspections are part of the regular program of inspections and can be **initial inspections** or **subsequent inspections**. Those initial or subsequent inspections found in full compliance (NAI—no action indicated) or with minor deficiencies (VAI—voluntary action indicated) usually will be assigned for reinspection within the following 5 years to determine their continued compliance with the regulations. Those found with serious violations (OAI— official action indicated) of the regulations will usually be assigned reinspection within 1 year to confirm that adequate corrections have been made.

2. *Directed.* A directed inspection may be assigned when the FDA receives information that puts into question the IRB practices and procedures. A directed inspection may be partial, limited to the area of concern, or may cover the entire compliance program.

3.10 WHAT TO DO WHEN AN IRB FDA INSPECTION IS ANNOUNCED

Tip: Do Not Panic!

Normally, the FDA's district offices (the inspector) will contact a responsible individual at the institution, usually the IRB chairperson, to schedule the site visit. The site inspection should occur within 10 days of the announcement. It is recommended that the IRB chairperson enquire about the scope of the inspection in order to focus on the documents that the IRB has to prepare for the inspection.

1. After the inspection is announced, the IRB chairperson should notify all IRB members of the impending inspection, along with the CEO and any other relevant party within the institution.

2. The IRB chairperson should inform all investigators of the institution of the upcoming inspection.

3. The IRB chairperson should also make provisions for a place where the inspection will take place. It is recommended that a meeting room is reserved for that purpose with access to a phone and copying services. **Do not use the IRB filing room for the inspection**. The IRB must ensure that there is a responsible person who will accompany the inspector at all times and photocopy all materials requested by the inspectors **personally**. At that time, a **second copy** must be generated should an observation arise for the IRB.

4. The IRB should preinspect all documentation and SOPs according to the FDA recommended checklist.

5. The IRB chairperson must ensure that all documentation on site or archived is available should the inspector request it.

6. If the IRB was previously inspected, follow-up on Form 483 if any was issued, the correspondence and outcome.

7. The IRB should prepare the documentation listed in Table 3.7.

According to FDA guidelines, the studies selected for FDA inspection should represent current IRB practices, preferably studies approved within the previous 3 years, and they should be chosen according to the following priority:

1. Safety and efficacy studies of investigational new drugs, devices, and/or biologics performed under an IND or IDE.

2. Comparison studies of one or more marketed products with an investigational one.

3. Studies for which no FDA research permit is required, as are certain marketed drugs and nonsignificant risk devices.

The IRB should follow the same priority in the preinspection and organization of documents.

TABLE 3.7 Documentation for an Inspection of an Institutional Review Board

Documents related to the submitted studies
  by the investigators as are:

Protocols and amendments reviewed
  Informed consent forms
  Investigator's Brochures
  Other documentation provided
    to patients
  Media ads

The Standard operating procedures according
  to the FDA Evaluation Checklist for IRB
All SAEs submitted by sponsors and
  investigators and follow-ups
IRB authorities (names of chairperson,
  secretary, etc.) and organizational chart

Documents related to the studies sent by the
  IRB to the clinical investigator as are:

Letters of refusal, approval, request for
  more information, re-approval after
  continuous review

List of all studies reviewed
Minutes of meetings

List of IRB members and their occupations

3.11 THE INVESTIGATOR SITE INSPECTION

The FDA inspector will audit the investigator site according to the responsibilities that the investigator assumed (or should have assumed) by signing Form 1572—Statement of the Investigator). Additionally, the FDA establishes the investigator's responsibilities to conduct clinical investigations for FDA-regulated products and every investigator should be aware of those responsibilities before agreeing to participate in a clinical study.

3.11.1 Objective of an FDA Investigator Site Inspection

The FDA conducts clinical investigator inspections to determine if the clinical investigators are operating in compliance with current FDA regulations and statutory requirements. Clinical investigators who conduct FDA-regulated clinical investigations are required to permit FDA investigators to access, copy, and verify any records or reports made by the clinical investigator with regard to the disposition of the product and subject case histories (21 CFR 312.68 and 812.145).

Clinical investigators are required to retain records for a period of 2 years following the date a marketing application is approved for the product or, if no application is filed or if the application is not approved, until 2 years after the investigation is discontinued and the FDA is notified. (See 21 CFR 312.62(c) and 812.140.)

3.11.2   Dynamics of a Clinical Investigator's Inspection (Scope)

The inspection will involve the comparison of the practices and procedures of the clinical investigator with the commitments made in the applicable regulations as described in Chapter 48, Bioresearch Monitoring Program CP 7648.811. These inspections include factual comparison of data submitted to the sponsor with supporting data in the clinical investigator's file (source data).

3.12   INVESTIGATOR'S RESPONSIBILITIES

The FDA regulations governing the conduct of clinical trials by clinical investigators are intended to assure adequate protection of the rights, safety, and welfare of subjects involved in those trials, as well as the quality and integrity of the resulting data.

These responsibilities are assumed by the investigator of a clinical trial or are implicit when conducting investigational testing in human subjects.

These responsibilities apply to any person who conducts a clinical investigation of a drug, biologic, or medical device [an investigator as defined in 21 CFR 312.3(b) and 21 CFR 812.3(i) and 21 CFR 312.60, 21 CFR Parts 50 and 56].

The responsibilities of an investigator are defined in the Code of Federal Regulations.

1. *Investigators must assure that an Institutional Review Board (IRB) that complies with FDA regulations conducts initial and continuing ethical review of the study (21 CFR Part 56 and § 312.66).* The investigator must therefore be knowledgeable of the requirements for a duly constituted IRB and should obtain written procedures of that IRB together with the inspectional history, if any are available. As stated before, a noncompliant IRB's approval is equivalent to the investigators and sponsor as not having any approval at all. Also, the investigator should be aware that as of July 14, 2009 the FDA requires IRBs to register through a system maintained by the Department of Health and Human Services (HHS). The registration information includes contact information (such as addresses and telephone numbers), the number of active protocols involving FDA-regulated products reviewed during the preceding 12 months, and a description of the types of FDA-regulated products involved in the protocols reviewed. The IRB registration requirements will make it easier for the FDA to inspect IRBs and to convey information to IRBs.

2. *An investigator must notify the IRB of changes in the research activity or unanticipated problems involving risks to human subjects or others, and must not make any changes in the protocol without IRB and sponsor approval, unless necessary to eliminate apparent immediate hazards to human subjects (21 CFR 312.66).* There should be an open communication between the IRB and the investigator, and at the same time the IRB should act promptly on requests of review for changes or amendments to protocols. The investigator

must know the processes and procedures of their IRBs and submit documents for review in a expedite manner.

3. *An investigator must also obtain informed consent from each subject who participates in the study (21 CFR 312.60 and 21 CFR Part 50).* The investigator should first obtain IRB approval of the Patient Information and Consent Form. Only the approved form should be utilized, and consent should be obtained prior to any clinical trial activity, including gathering of data from the patient for trial purposes.

The investigator is responsible for obtaining consent. However, that responsibility of explaining and signing the consent form can be delegated, in writing according to specified procedures, to a person who is qualified to obtain consent. Then there should be a procedure and a document to provide assurance that the investigator acknowledges that a duly signed consent was obtained prior to the subject's participation in a trial.

4. *In signing Form 1572 the investigator agrees to the following:*

(a) To conduct the study(ies) in accordance with the relevant, current protocol(s) (protocol adherence) and to only make changes in a protocol after notifying the sponsor, except when necessary to protect the safety, rights, or welfare of subjects;

It is very important that investigators understand the significance of protocol adherence to be able to comprehend the consequences. First, when a protocol is approved by the regulator and the IRB, this means that all possible precautions and measures have been taken within the regulations to ensure patient's safety. Changes of protocol procedures without an in-depth analysis of the consequences of those changes by the parties may shift the risk-benefit assessment previously conducted to unacceptable levels. In addition, clinical trials are now conducted at more than one site, actually they are global. Therefore, we need consensus with the investigators that all will follow the same protocol procedures as described. Clinical trials are in essence controlled experimentation in human subjects to demonstrate a hypothesis. All the elements of the control must be met to have the data qualify for statistical analysis. Changes in assessment type, frequency, schedule, and/or treatments may render data impossible to analyze and therefore the investigator may have introduced an incredible number of variables previously not defined, and therefore the result may not have any statistical or clinical significance.

Therefore, adherence to the protocol will provide a degree of assurance on patient safety and data credibility.

(b) To personally conduct or supervise the described investigation(s).

This is a very important responsibility that investigators fail to recognize and therefore may be construed as noncompliant. The FDA identifies that any investigator who conducts clinical investigations of drugs, including biological products, under 21 CFR Part 312 commits to personally conduct or supervise the investigation. Investigators who conduct clinical investigations of medical devices, under 21 CFR Part 812, commit to supervising all testing of the device involving human subjects.

Since clinical trials are very complex and time consuming, investigators may need assistance to meet the time requirements for completing studies. Therefore, it was recognized as common practice for investigators to delegate certain study-related tasks to employees, colleagues, or other third parties (individuals or entities not under the direct supervision of the investigator).

When tasks are delegated by the investigator, **the investigator is responsible for providing adequate supervision of those to whom tasks are delegated and the investigator is accountable for regulatory violations resulting from failure to adequately supervise the conduct of the clinical study.**

During an inspection of an investigational site, the FDA will focus on four major issues (FDA-Guidance for Industry Investigator Responsibilities: Protecting the Rights, Safety, and Welfare of Study Subjects, October 2009):

(i) **Whether delegated individuals were qualified to perform such tasks,** by training and experience, or, if a medical task, by licensing and practice.

(ii) **Whether study staff received adequate training on how to conduct the delegated tasks and were provided with an adequate understanding of the study**. Usually, in clinical trials the principal investigator will receive training through investigator meetings on the study protocol and study procedures. The training will be documented and the investigator will be considered qualified. The investigator must ensure that the information is appropriately relayed to all personnel involved in the study. However, in many cases, subinvestigators perform certain activities such as assessing patients for eligibility and applying a scale or inclusion/exclusion criteria. Unless there is written evidence that the subinvestigator is qualified by training, background, experience, and qualifications as well as licensure requirements as stated in the protocol, that person may not be "qualified" in the eyes of the regulator to perform such activities, and moreover may not have any records of training in the study protocol.

Note that the investigator should maintain a list of the appropriately qualified persons to whom significant trial-related duties have been delegated as required by GCP. This list should also describe the delegated tasks, identify the training that individuals have received that qualifies them to perform delegated tasks, and identify the dates of involvement in the study. An investigator should maintain separate lists for each study conducted by the investigator.

Adequate training is a very broad concept unless specified as follows:

- Have a general familiarity with the study and the protocol
- Have a specific understanding of the details of the protocol and the investigational product, relevant to the tasks to be performed
- Are aware of regulatory requirements and acceptable standards for the conduct of clinical trials, with respect to both the conduct of the clinical trial and human subject protection

- Are competent to perform the tasks that they are delegated
- Are informed of any pertinent changes during the conduct of the trial and educated or given additional training as appropriate

(iii) **Whether there is adequate supervision of the conduct of an ongoing clinical trial.** Having the investigator delegate some activities to study personnel **does not** imply that the responsibilities were also delegated. The investigator retains the responsibility for those activities and therefore must supervise all their personnel adequately.

The investigator should have sufficient time to properly conduct and supervise the clinical trial.

The FDA considers that supervision and oversight should be provided even for individuals who are highly qualified and experienced. A supervision plan might include the following elements, to the extent that they apply to a particular trial:

- Routine meetings with staff to review trial progress and update staff on any changes to the protocol or other procedures
- Routine meetings with the sponsor's monitors
- A procedure for correcting problems identified by study personnel, outside monitors or auditors, or other parties involved in the conduct of a study
- A procedure for documenting the performance of delegated tasks in a satisfactory manner and, where appropriate, verifying findings (e.g., observation of the performance of selected assessments or independent verification by repeating selected assessments)
- A procedure for ensuring that the consent process is being conducted in accordance with 21 CFR Part 50 and that study subjects understand the nature of their participation, risks, and so on.
- A procedure for ensuring that information in source documents is accurately captured on the Case Report Forms
- A procedure for dealing with data queries and discrepancies identified by the study monitor
- Procedures for ensuring study staff comply with the protocol, adverse event assessment and reporting, and other medical issues that arise during the course of the study

(iv) **Investigator's responsibilities for oversight of other parties involved in the conduct of a clinical trial.** Third parties may involve clinical trial site personnel provided by a site management organization (SMO). As previously mentioned, these organizations, unless they provide a service to the sponsor of a clinical trial, are not recognized under the regulations as CROs. Therefore, it is the responsibility of the investigator to oversee any activity performed by personnel of the SMO assigned to the site. The investigator should have processes implemented to ensure that the activities are conducted according to the protocol and regulatory requirements and take all necessary steps to assure compliance.

Parties other than the study staff. The FDA has identified that there are other third parties providing services to the study site directly or indirectly. In the case when central laboratory facilities are utilized to perform safety testing such as ECG or EEG, and clinical laboratory testing, the results are relayed directly to the sponsor and the investigator. The sponsor, having contracted those services (e.g., a central laboratory), seems to be directly responsible for the quality of the service and data provided; therefore, the investigator should not be involved in directly supervising those activities.

However, when services are contracted directly by the investigator with a third party facility (e.g., local laboratories) to provide for safety data for the clinical study, the FDA has identified the investigator as the responsible party to assure for the quality and integrity of those data and therefore the investigator must take steps to demonstrate oversight (obtain certifications of the facilities and qualifications of the personnel).

In any of the cases presented, the investigator should ensure data accuracy and credibility from third party providers and therefore carefully review the reports from external sources for results that are inconsistent with clinical presentation. To the extent feasible, and considering the specifics of study design, the clinical investigator should evaluate whether results appear reasonable, individually and in aggregate. If clinical investigators detect possible errors or suspect that results from a central laboratory might be questionable, the investigator should contact the sponsor immediately.

Specialized oversight in device studies or study data processing hardware. In some cases, specialized expertise from a device sponsor is needed to perform certain tasks. For example, when there is no one at the clinical site who can program an investigational pacemaker, the expertise may be provided by the sponsor's personnel, such as a field clinical engineer. The field clinical engineer should be supervised by the sponsor and not by the clinical investigator. When a field clinical engineer is designated by the sponsor to perform a specific activity within the investigational plan, this activity should be described in the protocol. **The investigator retains responsibility for ensuring that the protocol is followed**.

In the case where the sponsor provides for **study data processing hardware,** the investigator must ensure that all personnel using the equipment are trained to do so; however, the sponsor is responsible for providing for maintenance and upgrade of the systems if required. The investigator should retain all documentation that the activity took place according to the protocol and regulatory requirements.

(c) Protecting the Rights, Safety, and Welfare of Study Subjects.

As discussed previously, the Declaration of Helsinki is one of the main documents that states responsibilities of investigators for protecting the rights, safety, and well-being of subjects under their care. The FDA makes clear that clinical investigators are indeed responsible for protecting the rights, safety, and welfare of subjects under their care during a clinical trial (21 CFR 312.60 and 812.100).

(i) The FDA establishes that **reasonable medical care necessitated** by participation in a clinical trial should be provided by the investigator. That applies to the periods during and after the study is completed. Either that care should be provided by the investigator or the subject should be referred to a physician specialist to treat a particular condition.

(ii) Medical care should be provided in the case where a subject experiences any adverse events, including clinically significant laboratory values, related to the trial.

(iii) Far beyond the objectives of the study, the investigator should inform a subject when medical care is needed for intercurrent illness(es).

(iv) If the subject has a primary physician and agrees to the primary physician being informed, the investigator should inform the subject's primary physician about the subject's participation in the trial.

(v) Subjects should receive appropriate medical evaluation and treatment until resolution of **any condition related to the study intervention that develops during the course of their participation in a study,** even if the follow-up period extends beyond the end of the study at the investigative site. Although this point does not discuss in detail the financial implication of having to provide medical care to a subject who participates in a clinical study and develops a trial-related adverse event, the investigator must ensure that the right to access care is not violated by the financial burden to which a patient may be subjected if the financial aspects are not clearly established. These aspects should be clearly detailed in the Patient Information and Consent Form.

(vi) Subjects should have reasonable access to medical care. When an investigator agrees to be the principal investigator for a clinical trial, he/she assumes all required responsibilities, including providing reasonable access to medical care for subjects in a study. Regardless of the interpretation of this requirement, a patient should have access to qualified medical care at all times during the study. This means that the principal investigator or delegate (identified in Form 1572 as a subinvestigator) assumes the responsibility of being available at the site in a reasonable time, or by phone or other way, to assist a subject who may be in need of care. The delegation should be properly documented and also submitted to the IRB for review.

(vii) Protocol violations that present unreasonable risks must be avoided. Clinical investigators are required to comply with protocol procedures since those were established to protect the rights, safety, and warfare of subjects. The investigator must therefore be very familiar with the protocol and procedures to identify the critical points. The investigator should not deviate from protocol procedures (e.g., safety assessments) because patients may be subjected to unnecessary risk. For example, failure to adhere to inclusion/exclusion criteria that are specifically intended to exclude subjects for whom the study drug or device poses unreasonable risks (e.g., enrolling a subject with decreased renal function in a trial in which decreased function is exclusionary because the drug may be nephrotoxic) may be considered failure to protect the rights, safety, and welfare of the enrolled subject.

In summary, by signing Form 1572, the investigator agrees to the following:

COMMITMENTS:

I agree to conduct the study(ies) in accordance with the relevant, current protocol(s) and will only make changes in a protocol after notifying the sponsor, except when necessary to protect the safety, rights, or welfare of subjects.

I agree to personally conduct or supervise the described investigation(s).

I agree to inform any patients, or any persons used as controls, that the drugs are being used for investigational purposes and I will ensure that the requirements relating to obtaining informed consent in 21 CFR Part 50 and institutional review board (IRB) review and approval in 21 CFR Part 56 are met.

I agree to report to the sponsor adverse experiences that occur in the course of the investigation(s) in accordance with 21 CFR 312.64.

I have read and understand the information in the investigator's brochure, including the potential risks and side effects of the drug.

I agree to ensure that all associates, colleagues, and employees assisting in the conduct of the study(ies) are informed about their obligations in meeting the above commitments.

I agree to maintain adequate and accurate records in accordance with 21 CFR 312.62 and to make those records available for inspection in accordance with 21 CFR 312.68.

I will ensure that an IRB that complies with the requirements of 21 CFR Part 56 will be responsible for the initial and continuing review and approval of the clinical investigation. I also agree to promptly report to the IRB all changes in the research activity and all unanticipated problems involving risks to human subjects or others. Additionally, I will not make any changes in the research without IRB approval, except where necessary to eliminate apparent immediate hazards to human subjects.

And remember that the investigator also agrees to the following:

I agree to comply with all other requirements regarding the obligations of clinical investigators and all other pertinent requirements in 21 CFR Part 312.

Compliance to 21 CFR 312.60 entitles, for instance, the following:

An investigator is responsible for ensuring that an investigation is conducted according to:

- The signed investigator statement (Form 1572), the investigational plan, and applicable regulations; for protecting the rights, safety, and welfare of subjects under the investigator's care; and

- For the control of drugs under investigation (Sec. 312.61). An investigator shall administer the drug **only to subjects under the investigator's personal supervision or under the supervision of a sub investigator responsible to the investigator.** The investigator shall not supply the investigational drug to any person not authorized under this part to receive it.

- An investigator shall, in accordance with the provisions of part 50 of this chapter, **obtain the informed consent of each human subject to whom the drug is administered,** except as provided in 50.23 or 50.24 of this chapter. (Additional specific responsibilities of clinical investigators are set forth in this part and in parts 50 and 56 of this chapter.)

- **Investigator recordkeeping and record retention Sec. 312.62.**

  (a) *Disposition of drug.* An investigator is required to maintain adequate records of the disposition of the drug, including dates, quantity, and use by subjects. If the investigation is terminated, suspended, discontinued, or completed, the investigator shall return the unused supplies of the drug to the sponsor, or otherwise provide for disposition of the unused supplies of the drug under 312.59.

  (b) *Case histories.* An investigator is required to prepare and maintain adequate and accurate case histories that record all observations and other data pertinent to the investigation on each individual administered the investigational drug or employed as a control in the investigation. Case histories include the case report forms and supporting data including, for example, signed and dated consent forms and medical records, including progress notes of the physician, the individual's hospital chart(s), and the nurses' notes. The case history for each individual shall document that informed consent was obtained prior to participation in the study. This means that the investigator MUST make a note in the patient file/case history that the consent was obtained.

  (c) *Record retention.* An investigator shall retain records required to be maintained under this part for a period of 2 years following the date a marketing application is approved for the drug for the indication for which it is being investigated; or, if no application is to be filed or if the application is not approved for such indication, until 2 years after the investigation is discontinued and FDA is notified. (in other countries may be longer as in Canada is for 25 years)

- **Investigator reports Sec. 312.64**

  (a) *Progress reports.* The investigator shall furnish all reports to the sponsor of the drug who is responsible for collecting and evaluating the results obtained. The sponsor is required under 312.33 to submit annual reports to FDA on the progress of the clinical investigations.

(**b**) *Safety reports.* An investigator shall promptly report to the sponsor any adverse effect that may reasonably be regarded as caused by, or probably caused by, the drug. If the adverse effect is alarming, the investigator shall report the adverse effect immediately.

(**c**) *Final report.* An investigator shall provide the sponsor with an adequate report shortly after completion of the investigator's participation in the investigation.

(**d**) *Financial disclosure reports.* The clinical investigator shall provide the sponsor with sufficient accurate financial information to allow an applicant (this is the sponsor) to submit complete and accurate certification or disclosure statements as required under 21 CFR part 54. The clinical investigator shall promptly update this information if any relevant changes occur during the course of the investigation and for 1 year following the completion of the study.

- **Assurance of IRB review Sec. 312.66**
  An investigator shall assure that an IRB that complies with the requirements set forth in part 56 will be responsible for the initial and continuing review and approval of the proposed clinical study. Also, that the IRB is registered with the FDA by July 14, 2009 (21 CFR 56.106(a)). The investigator shall also assure that he or she will promptly report to the IRB all changes in the research activity and all unanticipated problems involving risk to human subjects or others, and that he or she will not make any changes in the research without IRB approval, except where necessary to eliminate apparent immediate hazards to human subjects.

- **Inspection of investigator's records and reports Sec. 312.68**
  An investigator shall upon request from any properly authorized officer or employee of FDA, at reasonable times, permit such officer or employee to have access to, and copy and verify any records or reports made by the investigator pursuant to 312.62. The investigator is not required to divulge subject names unless the records of particular individuals require a more detailed study of the cases, or unless there is reason to believe that the records do not represent actual case studies, or do not represent actual results obtained.

- **Handling of controlled substances Sec. 312.69**
  If the investigational drug is subject to the Controlled Substances Act, the investigator shall take adequate precautions, including storage of the investigational drug in a securely locked, substantially constructed cabinet, or other securely locked, substantially constructed enclosure, access to which is limited, to prevent theft or diversion of the substance into illegal channels of distribution.

3.13 TYPES OF CLINICAL INVESTIGATOR SITE INSPECTIONS

The clinical investigator inspection program includes the following types of inspections:

1. **Study-Oriented Inspections**. Assignments are based almost exclusively on studies that are important to product evaluation, such as new drug applications

and product license applications. These are regular inspections conducted after an NDA was submitted.

2. **Investigator-Oriented Inspections**. This type of inspection is based more on issues pertaining to a particular investigator than study.

   - The FDA may consider the site because the investigator conducted a pivotal study.
   - The sponsor may have reported to the FDA that there are concerns about the investigator's work.
   - The FDA may initiate an inspection, if a subject in a study complains about protocol or subject rights violations.
   - The clinical investigator may have participated in a large number of studies or have done work outside his/her specialty areas.
   - The safety or effectiveness findings at that site are inconsistent with those of other investigators.

3. **Bioequivalence Study Inspections**. Bioequivalence study inspections are conducted because one study may be the sole basis for a (i.e., generic) drug's marketing approval. The bioequivalence study inspection differs from the other inspections in that it requires participation by an FDA chemist or an investigator knowledgeable about analytical evaluations to assist the inspection.

3.14   INSPECTIONAL PROCEDURES

3.14.1   The Investigator Site Documentation and Organization

Once the objective of an investigator site audit or inspection is established, the focus will be shifted to the process itself.

The regulatory inspector can only perform an audit according to the documentation available at the site, comparing those documents to the data submitted by the sponsor and the commitments assumed by the investigator.

The investigator is required to maintain adequate records of the studies conducted (Sec. 312.62.) and retain them accordingly. The investigator should have a filing system similar to the sponsor's Trial Master File for each and every study conducted. All the documentation should be legible, not only clean and neat, but in the language of the inspector. Illegible documents should be retyped and/or translated before the inspector comes to allow easy access to information, and both copies should be available for inspection.

All the essential documents for a clinical trial as stated in GCP will be inspected together with regulatory documents. Therefore, the site should prepare all documents as described in the Table 3.4.

Source documents should be clearly identified and requested by the investigator site ahead of time if they are filed in a central filing system.

3.14.2 The Sponsor's Role in the Investigator Site Audit

The investigator should promptly notify the sponsor of an impending inspection. It is very important since the sponsor may assist the site with a preinspection to verify that all documentation and materials are available for the regulatory inspector. Also, the sponsor may provide for regulatory support before, during, and after the inspection. Although sponsors might not be directly involved in regulatory site inspections, the sponsor's data validity and quality are being scrutinized, therefore the sponsor's involvement should be significant.

Also remember to notify the institution if you are located within a health or research facility.

3.14.3 The Clinical Investigator Site Inspection Step by Step: The Day of the Inspection

Prepare all the personnel at the site to receive the inspector since all personnel can and will be interviewed briefly. Explain to the clinical trial site personnel the purpose and scope of the inspection from what was relayed to the investigator during the phone call or from Form 482 announcing the inspector's visit. Have your personnel arrive at least one hour earlier to prepare all details before the inspector arrives. Check that all documents are available and organize them on the desk according to a system that will allow easy access. Make sure that all documents are available. (See Table 3.8.)

When the inspector arrives he/she will introduce him/herself and the accompanying team to the assigned greeter who was particularly chosen by the principal investigator.

Make sure that the FDA inspector presents a photo ID, and take note of the name and ID number.

Upon arrival and identification, you should take the inspector to the area you have assigned to the inspector (and team) and where the documents are located. Make sure this is adequate. Adequacy means that it is a clean room with a desk and chairs, phone, power jacks for the computers, and wireless access to the Internet (although not necessary). It is also better if the room has a window.

TABLE 3.8 To Do List the Day of the Inspection Before Inspector Arrives

Item	Action
1	Prepare all the personnel at the site to receive the inspector since all personnel can and will be interviewed briefly.
2	Explain to the clinical trial site personnel the purpose and scope of the inspection from what was relayed to the investigator during the phone call announcing the inspector's visit.
3	Have your personnel arrive one hour earlier to prepare all details before the inspector arrives.
4	Check that all documents are available and organize them on the desk according to a system that will allow easy access.
5	Assign a person who will greet the inspector(s).

At that point the inspector should present you with the Notice of Inspection (FDA Form 482) where the scope and objective of the inspection are detailed. A copy of that form should be filed in the Investigators File for future reference.

Following this, the inspector(s) may want to inspect the facilities where the study took place and interview the personnel who may have participated in the study. Provide ample time for that purpose.

It is very important that the clinical investigator adjusts all his/her activities on the day of the inspection to allow ample time to take part in the inspection, and that the facilities inspection itself does not interfere with other previously planned tasks for the site.

3.15 FDA AUDIT PROCEDURES FOR INVESTIGATIVE SITES

3.15.1 Authority and Administration

It is very important that you prepare the answers to the questions that customarily are put forth by an inspector ahead of time to allow a smooth interaction. Also, practice with your team on the most important issues.

Note that the FDA has established policies on refusals to provide information or documents. If during the inspection, access to records or copying of records is refused for any reason or there is what is called a de facto refusal, the FDA investigator will immediately report to his/her superiors, which may prompt additional actions. If the investigator site does not have the documentation requested for any reason (e.g., as lost, misplaced, or never obtained) do not refuse to provide it: explain that the document was lost or misplaced and make all efforts to find it while the inspector is at the site.

Many investigators may feel uneasy to provide access to patient files in light of confidentiality of medical records; however, the investigator must recall that when he/she signed Form 1572, he/she agreed to provide all records or reports to the inspector and that the patient files are part of those records.

During the establishment inspection, the inspector may interview the personnel to verify the following activities:

1. *Who Did What?* Who performed the various clinical trial activities, such as who obtained informed consent, who verified inclusion and exclusion criteria, and who collected adverse event data. Have prepared an organizational chart, with the main activities.

2. *Delegation of authority*

   (a) How the clinical investigator supervised the conduct of the investigation. Have available minutes of internal meetings and principal investigator's notes and follow-ups.

(b) Determine whether authority for the conduct of the various aspects of the study was delegated properly so that the investigator retained control and knowledge of the study. Have available the procedure for delegation of authority and the documents delegating responsibilities to the various parties, such as contract agreements or delegation letters.

3. *Specific Site of Study Activities.* Where specific aspects of the investigation were performed: like logs, charts, appointment schedules, and lab requisitions and results.

4. *Data Recording.* How and where data were recorded. Have available the patient files or charts as well as the consent forms and case report forms.

5. *Drug Accountability.* Accountability for the investigational product. Have all updated drug accountability logs available.

6. *Monitoring*

(a) The monitor's communications with the clinical investigator, such as emails, letters, and other communications.

(b) The monitor's evaluations of the progress of the investigation, such as progress letters or reports.

(c) Determine how (e.g., telephone, memo, etc.) the monitor explained to the clinical investigator the status of the test article, nature of the protocol, and the obligations of a clinical investigator. Depending on the sponsor, this may be through a verbal interview or a follow-up letter after the monitoring visit.

7. *Investigator's Supervision*

(a) Whether there was adequate supervision and involvement in the ongoing conduct of the study. This refers to documents showing the investigator's involvement (such as visit reports, follow-ups and minutes of meetings conducted with clinical trial personnel).

(b) Whether there was adequate supervision or oversight of any third parties involved in the conduct of a study (contractors, CROs) to the extent that such supervision or oversight was reasonably possible. This will depend on the activity contracted; however, the investigator must have an answer as to how he/she supervised the activity.

8. The FDA inspector will also try to determine whether the investigator discontinued the study before completion.

9. The FDA inspector will request a list of the names and addresss of the facility(ies) performing laboratory tests.

(a) If any laboratory testing was performed in the investigator's own facility, determine whether that facility is equipped to perform each test specified. This refers to certificates of accreditation accrediting the facility for the time the study took place or is taking place.

(b) List the name(s) of individuals performing such tests and indicate their position. This list should also include licenses that the personnel may have to hold to perform specific activities (such as a licensed pathologist).

3.15.2   Inspecting the Protocol

The clinical trial site should prepare all the IRB approved versions of the protocol and amendments utilized during the inspected study together with the IRB approval letters and notifications.

The inspector will require the following:

1. Copies of the protocol and all IRB approvals and modifications (including the version numbers and effective dates) to the protocol. If a copy is not available, such will be immediately reported. Therefore, request a new copy from the sponsor if you lost it.

2. The inspector will compare the copies at the site with the ones provided previously by the sponsor and forwarded by the regional office. *Note: The copies must be IDENTICAL.* To compare the versions presented to what was submitted, the inspector will compare the following: (a) subject selection (i.e., inclusion and exclusion criteria), (b) number of subjects, (c) frequency of subject observations, (d) dosage, (e) route of administration, (f) frequency of dosage, (g) blinding procedures, and (h) other, such as specific aspects of the study.

3. The inspector will determine whether all changes to the protocol were (a) documented by an approved amendment, (b) dated, (c) maintained with the protocol, and (d) approved by the IRB and reported to the sponsor before implementation and, except where necessary, to eliminate apparent immediate hazard to human subjects.

Note that the *Compliance Program Guidance Manual for FDA Staff* (Compliance Program 7348.811-Part III) states clearly that deviations from the protocol are not to be interpreted as changes, and therefore should not be identified as such.

3.15.3   Inspecting Subjects' Records

The inspector, by comparing of practices and procedures, will check for data credibility and integrity. For that purpose the investigator should prepare all subject records for the identified subject by the inspector.

Those records include the source documents such as the patient files, charts, exam results, and others. The inspector will determine the following:

1. **Organization, Condition, Completeness, and Legibility of the Records Presented.** All records must follow an organizational structure, and access should be simple. All records presented must be legible, not only the print, but the language in which they were written. If the language is other than that spoken by the inspectors, make sure that the records are properly translated. If the records are old and the writing is dim (done in pencil or printed on thermal paper), make sure that those records have a photocopy done before filing or archiving, and make every effort to ensure legibility at all times (avoid coffee spills and other stains that may obscure the original information).

2. **Whether There Is Adequate Documentation to Assure that All Audited Subjects Did Exist and Were Alive and Available for the Duration of Their**

Stated Participation in the Study. It is very important to remember that fraud is a serious offence in any circumstance. The investigator should make an effort to **only enroll patients who can demonstrate existence and availability**. That is a key reason for enrolling only citizens of the United States or legal aliens for whom traceability is possible, if necessary.

3. **Compare the Source Documents in the Clinical Investigator's Records with the Case Report Forms Completed for the Sponsor**. Determine whether clinical laboratory testing (including EKGs, X rays, eye exams, etc.), as noted in the case report forms, was documented by the presence of completed laboratory records among the source documents. The inspector will check each critical field in the CRF against data at the source, and he/she will work backwards starting form the information provided by the sponsor in the market application for that site and comparing it to the patient files and laboratory results. If inconsistencies are found, the inspector may widen the scope of the inspection. Remember that data should correspond 100%. Inconsistencies in data collection and transfer as well as errors will be seen as monitoring or quality assurance concerns that may involve the sponsor in the expanded scope of an audit.

4. **Whether All Adverse Experiences Were Reported in the Case Report Forms**. Not reported or underreported adverse events are key findings in inspections. The safety profile of a product may be skewed if the reporting is not consistent. It is important to indicate that during monitoring of the site the monitor was able to identify all adverse experiences as established in the protocol. Also, it is important to note the "medical opinion" of the investigator regarding an experience in classifying it as serious or not. The sponsor has the responsibility to clarify the matter and document it in the form of a letter to the investigator or other report, before an inspection brings it up.

5. **Whether Adverse Experiences Were Regarded as Caused by or Associated with the Test Article and If They Were Previously Anticipated (Specificity and Severity) in Any Written Information Regarding the Test Article**. The inspector will assess the adverse experiences according to the protocol and Investigator's Brochure, and if serious adverse experiences are evident, he/she will determine if there is information regarding relationship to the investigational product and if they were previously described. Here it is important to clarify that a change in severity and intensity of a previously described adverse event may render it reportable as an unexpected serious adverse event, and the investigator should have clear guidance from the sponsor as to when to report. Issues may arise regarding the "medical opinion" of the investigator and the classification of the adverse event. Therefore is important that the investigator site gather all information possible regarding all adverse events.

6. **Concomitant Therapy and/or Intercurrent Illnesses that Might Interfere with the Evaluation of the Effect of the Test Article**. The inspector will determine if concomitant therapy and/or intercurrent illnesses were included in the case report forms, and collected according to the protocol. This is also

an important point because eligibility and safety may depend on intercurrent illnesses and concomitant therapies.

7. **Whether the Number and Type of Subjects Entered into the Study Were Eligible.** The issue of eligibility is very important because patient recruitment is always a challenge, and the strict conditions of inclusion/exclusion may have a great impact on the study viability. The investigator should document all information regarding eligibility of each included patient as well as the reasons for exclusion of all excluded patients to demonstrate absence of bias in selection. Entering noneligible patients is a serious violation of the protocol and may subject a patient to unreasonable risk. It is also practical to keep a patient screening log for potential patients who, although deemed eligible in principle, did not meet inclusion criteria or did not agree to sign consent.

8. **Whether the Existence of the Condition for Which the Test Article Was Being Studied Is Documented by Notation Made Prior to the Initiation of the Study or by a Compatible History.** (The patient had the disease for which the product is intended to be studied, diagnosed prior to initiating the study.) This inspectional aspect provides the rationale as to why it is important that investigators have access to potentially eligible subjects to enroll in a study. Note that subjects enrolled "out on the street" without previous history of the disease documented in the file can be hard to demonstrate as eligible if scarce information on the condition is available.

9. **Whether Each Record Contains Information on the Condition of a Subject.**

   (a) Observations, information, and data on the condition of the subject at the time the subject entered into the clinical study. The patient file should contain the information on the disease history, and data to support eligibility. It is very useful for the investigator to have a "template" for each visit to record information on the patient visit according to the protocol schedule. The investigator must not record data directly in the CRF since if the source is unavailable, data cannot be source verified and therefore is not suitable for submission.

   (b) Records of exposure of the subject to the test article. Drug dispensing logs as well as drug accountability records should be available and complete for each patient in the study and they have to be consistent with the protocol dosage regimen and duration of treatment. Inconsistencies on drug accountability are very notable violations. Investigators have to demonstrate that they had control of the investigational product at all times and that only eligible patients were dispensed the test article.

   (c) Observations and data on the condition of the subject throughout participation in the investigation including results of laboratory tests, development of unrelated illness, and other factors that might alter the effects of the test article. The investigator should have a detailed description of the patient's condition in the patient file during the entire study as a source for data on safety of the investigational product.

(d) The identity of all persons and locations obtaining raw data or involved in the collection or analysis of such data. A clinical trial personnel list and their duties should be available at the beginning of the inspection to familiarize the inspector with site personnel.

(e) The clinical investigator reports of all dropouts, and the reasons therefore, to the sponsor. Dropouts are a serious matter in clinical trials. When a patient decides to discontinue participation in a study, the investigator should make every effort to know why. Dropouts may hide patients with adverse events who did not communicate the event to the investigator or could not deal with the event anymore (e.g., continuous diarrhea). On the other hand, patients may drop out due to lack of efficacy, another hidden adverse event. In that case, the patient may have decided that he/she cannot continue with the symptoms of the condition untreated. In those cases, the inspector will ask for all documentation to support the dropout or all efforts made to contact a patient.

3.15.4 Inspecting Other Study Records

Patient safety is a key objective in FDA inspections. The inspectors are instructed to review information in the clinical investigator's records that will be helpful in assessing any underreporting of adverse experiences by the sponsor to the FDA.

1. The inspector will compare data supplied by the sponsor to the FDA to the information submitted by the clinical investigator to the sponsor from the clinical investigator's files.

2. In addition, the clinical investigator's correspondence files will be used for the adverse reactions and deaths. The inspector is instructed to document any discrepancies found.

The information that the inspector will utilize to detect underreporting of adverse events is the following: (1) the total number of subjects entered into the study, (2) the total number of dropouts from the study (identified by subject number), (3) the number of assessable subjects and the number of unassessable subjects (the latter identified by subject number), and (4) the adverse experiences, including deaths (with subject number and a description of the adverse experience or cause of death).

3.15.5 Inspecting the Consent of Human Subjects

The inspector will request a copy of the actual consent form signed by patients and approved by the IRB.

1. The inspector will determine if the consent was obtained prior to any clinical trial procedure. If the consent form was signed the same date that the patient

entered the study, there should be a time stamp to determine that it was obtained prior to the start of the procedure.

2. The inspector will also review the consent form to determine if it complies with 21 CFR 50.

3. If a representative was used or the consent was obtained verbally, conformance will also be determined.

4. The inspector will also determine if the consent process was compliant and the patient had effective time to decide and no pressure or coercion of any type was utilized.

5. The person obtaining consent if other than the investigator should be qualified to do so; therefore the inspector may require evidence of qualification.

6. There could also be a request to demonstrate that the patients signing the consent form understood the study and the procedures and the investigator should be prepared to answer that question too.

3.15.6 Inspecting the Institutional Review Board Documentation

The investigator agreed on Form 1572 that he/she "will ensure that an IRB that complies with the requirements of 21 CFR Part 56 will be responsible for the initial and continuing review and approval of the clinical investigation" and that he/she would obtain approval prior to initiation of the study. The inspector will try to obtain evidence of that as follows:

1. *Identify the name, address, and chairperson of the IRB for the study.* All IRB documentation gathered by the investigator has to be available for inspection, including membership, composition, standard operating procedures, letters of approval, and other communications.

2. *Determine whether the investigator maintains copies of all reports submitted to the IRB and reports of all actions by the IRB.* All submissions to the IRB have to be presented to the inspector as well as all the responses.

3. *Determine the nature and frequency of periodic reports submitted to the IRB.* The inspector will need access to the standard operating procedures of the IRB to determine reporting requirements. Copies of those SOPs should be available.

4. *Did the investigator submit to and obtain IRB approval of the following before subjects were allowed to participate in the investigation?*
   (a) Protocol
   (b) Modifications (amendments) to the protocol
   (c) Report of prior investigations (the Investigator's Brochure)
   (d) Materials to obtain human subject consent (consent form)
   (e) Media ads for patient/subject recruitment

Letters of approval identifying the protocol title and the version, together with documents reviewed, should be available for inspection.

5. *Determine whether the investigator submitted a report to the IRB of all deaths, adverse experiences, and unanticipated problems involving risk to human subjects* (21 CFR 312.66). All safety reports, internal or external, generated to date for the IRB should be available for inspection.

6. *The inspector will try to determine if the investigator made unauthorized statements in promotional materials.* Did the investigator disseminate any promotional material or otherwise represent that the test article is safe and effective for the purpose for which it is under investigation? Therefore, copies of all promotional materials should be available for inspection.

7. *The inspector will try to determine if the investigator had the promotional materials approved by the IRB before use by answering the following question.* Were these promotional materials submitted to the IRB for review and approval before use? Therefore, copies of the approval letters stating the materials approved should be available.

3.15.7 Inspecting the Sponsor's Documentation and Communications at the Investigator Site

The inspector has to determine that there was effective communication between the sponsor and the investigator. For that purpose the following will be inspected:

1. *Copy of the letter indicating IRB approved study.* To determine whether the investigator communicated approval and provided a copy of the IRB approved consent form to the sponsor.

2. *All periodic reports.* If periodic reports were submitted to the sponsor on time.

3. *Serious adverse event reports.* To determine if and how the investigator submitted a report of all deaths and adverse reactions to the sponsor.

4. *Completed and submitted CRFs where intercurrent illness and/or concomitant therapy are reported.* To determine whether all intercurrent illness and/or concomitant therapy were reported to the sponsor.

5. *All completed and submitted CRFs.* To determine whether all case report forms on subjects were submitted to the sponsor shortly after completion.

6. *All completed and submitted CRFs of dropout patients.* To determine whether all dropouts and the reasons therefore, were reported to the sponsor.

7. *Monitoring signature logs, monitoring letters, and phone or other communication records with the monitor.* To determine if the sponsor monitored the progress of the study to assure that investigator obligations were fulfilled. The inspector has to determine the modality of monitoring describing the method (on-site visit, telephone, contract research organization, etc.) and the frequency of monitoring.

3.15.8   Inspecting the Investigational Product (Test Article Accountability)

The investigator has responsibility for the investigational product at the site. Access, dispensing, and accountability will be scrutinized in detail. The following documentation should be available for inspection:

1. *List of authorized personnel to handle and dispense investigational product, including their qualifications (e.g. subinvestigators, pharmacists).* To determine whether unqualified or unauthorized persons administered or dispensed the test article.

2. *Copies of Form 1571 (for sponsor–investigator) and Form 1572.* The names of the persons authorized to handle investigational product is going to be represented on those forms. The inspector will compare the Form 1572 that was submitted by the sponsor against the one at the site and if there are discrepancies in the personnel handling the investigational product, it will be noted in the report.

3. *All investigational product accountability records.* Those records should include, for verification, the following information: (a) receipt date(s) and quantity; (b) dates and quantity dispensed, identification, and numbers of subjects; (c) that distribution of the test article was limited to those subjects under the investigator's or subinvestigator's direct supervision (that only eligible patients were dispensed study medication); (d) whether the quantity, frequency, duration, and route of administration of the test article, as reported to the sponsor, were generally corroborated by raw data notations (in the logs or patient files); and (e) date(s) and quantity returned to the sponsor or alternate disposition, authorization for alternate disposition, and the actual disposition.

   Also, information on the batch/lot number and expiration or reanalysis date should be available for inspection.

The inspector will actually compare the amount of test article usage with the amount shipped and returned. If available, the inspector will account for the unused supplies—count pills!—and verify that blinding, identity, lot number, and package and labeling agree with other study records describing the test article (protocol and Investigator's Brochure).

   The inspector may collect a sample if discrepancies are observed between the described investigational product and the actual product at the site.

4. *Investigational product storage area conditions.* The investigator should make arrangements to allow the inspector access to the investigational product storage area, especially if it is stored in the pharmacy.

   (a) If the investigational product had special storage conditions, there should be the following documents to determine that the conditions were maintained: temperature, humidity, and light exposure logs (if applicable) with data recorded according to protocol requirements.

(b) If the investigational product is a controlled substance, it should be stored according to local requirements and under secure lock in a substantially constructed enclosure. The inspector will determine the appropriateness of the storage conditions as well as access privileges to determine who had access to the controlled substance.

5. *Last patient, last dose.* The inspector has to determine the date on which the last subject completed the study to perform the final accountability for the investigational product and disposition (according to protocol requirements):

(a) CRFs and enrollment logs should be available to determine such date.

(b) Return date of test article as to the date the investigator discontinued or completed his/her participation; the date the sponsor discontinued or terminated the investigation; or the date the FDA terminated the investigation.

3.15.9   Inspecting the Records Retention Process

The agreement signed by the investigator together with the written communications with the sponsor should discuss the records retention process and custody of records.

That agreement, together with any other arrangement, should be available for inspection to determine the following:

1. Who maintains custody of the required records and the means by which prompt access can be assured.

2. Whether the investigator notified the sponsor in writing regarding the custody of required records, if the investigator does not retain them.

3. Whether the records are retained for the specified time as follows: (a) 2 years following the date on which the test article is approved by the FDA for marketing for the purposes which were the subject of the clinical investigation; or (b) 2 years following the date on which the entire clinical investigation (not just the investigator's part in it) is terminated or discontinued by the sponsor.

3.15.10   Inspecting Electronic Records and Signatures

Records in electronic form that are created, modified, maintained, archived, retrieved, or transmitted under any records requirement set forth in agency regulations must comply with 21 CFR 11.

In the case that the clinical trial site has electronic systems handling data, additional expertise will be incorporated in the inspection to determine compliance.

The investigator should have the following documentation available for inspection to determine adherence to 21 CFR 11:

1. *Hardware and Software Source Documents.* Invoices of purchase or other documentation of source (e.g., lease, license agreements).

2. *Installation and Training Records.* The investigator should have installation and maintenance logs including the name of the persons performing the installation and their qualifications. Also, the investigator should have evidence of training for use of the software and hardware.

3. *Software and/or Hardware Change Records.* The investigator should have evidence that the same systems and software were used during the entire study. If any changes in the hardware and/or software occurred during the clinical trial, proper validation of the systems should be available to demonstrate equivalent performance and integrity.

4. *Maintenance and Upgrade Records.* Electronic systems may require maintenance and upgrade. The investigator should keep detailed records of maintenance of the systems. Also, any upgrade to the systems must be validated and documented.

5. *System Errors and Failures.* The investigator should have available for inspection an error log as well as system problem logs to demonstrate stability and reliability.

6. *Source of Data Entered in the Computer.* According to the protocol when electronic systems are utilized, there may be different approaches as to the data flow:

   (a) *Paper source.* Data is collected in paper records (patient files) and then "entered" into the electronic CRF. In this case, the source is the patient files, as in paper case report forms.

   (b) *Direct.* Data is directly entered into the electronic CRF (though validated biometric equipment or other form). In this case, the source is the original file created with the data collected electronically.

   In any case, for data entered in the electronic case report form, details have to be provided on who entered the data and when it was entered.

7. *Electronic Systems Access Privileges and Records.* The investigator should provide a list of personnel who have access privileges to the electronic systems as well as time stamped and signed records of access per event.

8. *Security Procedures to Avoid Unauthorized Access.* The investigator should have available all security procedures to provide access only to authorized personnel. Any attempt at unauthorized access should also be documented.

9. *Data Verification and Change.* The electronic systems utilized at the investigator site where data is collected should provide for data verification and correction. Specific procedures should define who changes data, who authorizes changes, and who verifies (the investigator at the site or other authorized party), and how an audit trail is generated to avoid erasure of the original information.

10. *Data Submission Records.* The site should have available procedures for data transmission to the sponsor (i.e., modem, network, fax, hard disk, floppy disk,

electronic transfer, mail, messenger, picked up) and, according to the modality, all provisions taken to avoid data being altered during transfer. For example, if the Internet is utilized to transfer data from the site to the sponsor, extra procedures should be set in place for safety and security.

11. *Data Resolution Records.* If errors are discovered by the sponsor, records of data correction requisition, authorization and change, and audit trail should be available.

12. *Copies of Electronic Data Submitted.* The sponsor should make provision for a copy of data entered electronically in the CRF to be on file at the site. That copy can be printed or electronic according to the established procedures.

3.15.11   Inspecting Device Studies

The FDA strategies to inspect a device study follow equivalent procedures as for drugs. The objectives are the same as stated in the program. However, the regulations for investigational devices (21 CFR 812) do not contain all the provisions of the drug regulations. There is **no requirement that Forms 1571 or 1572** be used but there is a **requirement for a signed investigator agreement**. The inspector of a device study will focus on the following issues:

1. Whether the clinical investigator has used the test articles under the emergency use provisions. If so, the inspector will determine if the clinical investigator has adequately complied with the guidance documents for emergency use.

2. If the clinical investigator is involved in any nonsignificant risk studies and, if so, provide a list of these studies and ascertain if they are being conducted in compliance with regulations (must have nonsignificant determination by IRB and IRB approval).

3. If the clinical investigator has been involved in any use of a custom device. If so, the inspector will determine compliance with 21 CFR 812 regulations.

4. If the clinical investigator has been involved in any studies using humanitarian devices as provided by 21 CFR Part 814. A humanitarian use device (HUD) is a device that is intended to benefit subjects by treating or diagnosing a disease or condition that affects or is manifested in fewer than 4 000 individuals in the United States annually. The inspector will determine whether IRB approval was properly obtained.

3.16   FDA INSPECTIONS OF INTERNATIONAL CLINICAL TRIAL SITES

The FDA inspectional strategy involves foreign clinical trial sites that provide data for market applications in the United States. The selected sites will be scrutinized according to their compliance to FDA requirements and Good Clinical Practice. The process and procedures are similar; however, the actions may vary.

3.17 THE AUDIT REPORT AND FORM 483

At the end of an inspection, FDA personnel will conduct an exit interview with the clinical investigator or his/her representative. At this point, the investigator has the opportunity to discuss the findings and to provide more documentation to support compliance. It is very important that the clinical trial site investigator has regulatory support to understand the findings and to provide for an appropriate response. That regulatory support should be provided by an expert consultant or the industry sponsor. At this interview, FDA personnel who conducted the inspection will review and discuss the findings from the inspection. If deficiencies are found, they are summarized in a written FDA Form 483 (Inspectional Observations) that is then issued to the clinical investigator or his/her representative.

It is very important that the findings are taken seriously, and appropriate responses are provided in a timely manner.

The investigator should carefully read Form 483 and assess all documentation that supports the findings. To answer a Form 483, the investigator should seek expert assistance to provide the right information to the FDA and avoid further action.

3.17.1 The Exit Interview

We will take you now from the moment the inspector finishes inspecting your site and Form 483 is handed to you.

You are discussing with the inspector the findings. Let see what you should *not* do. **Never answer**:

- *Sorry...* Sorry does not help anyone, because you have to assume your responsibilities when signing Form 1572.
- *I did not know*. As an investigator, you *should* know what you are doing and what is required from you. Regulatory requirements and the protocol must be adhered to at all times.
- *It is not my fault, I did not do it*. Well, basically it *is* your fault because you should be personally supervising if not conducting the clinical trial.
- *That is my coordinator's fault*. Again, it is the investigator who is responsible for all clinical trial activities at the site.
- *This is new to me*. It is true that many changes happened recently in the requirements for clinical trials (especially with electronic data handling, registrations, etc.); however, the investigator should keep him/herself updated and should not be caught by surprise.

- *"Mea culpa," yes it is my fault.* Do not assume fault until you consult with an expert on the particular issue. The regulator is not interested in assigning you fault but correcting any violations so they do not occur in the future.

- *I do not agree with your opinion.* It is very important that the clinical investigator or representative does not become argumentative with the inspector since the inspector may write his/her opinion on Form 483; however, the center will review the case and will reassess the findings with all the supportive documents. You always have the opportunity to express your side of the story in the written response to Form 483 to the district office.

- DO NOT PROVIDE UNSOLICITED INFORMATION: you may dig yourself in deeper.

Once you have discussed the findings, gather all information to respond to Form 483 properly and ask for assistance from the sponsor, if you are sponsored by a pharmaceutical company, or from an expert consultant.

The following is what you *should do* during the exit interview:

- Be available for the interview.

- Listen carefully to the inspector, and take notes of his/her comments (those may be part of the internal report).

- Answer only if you really know what are you talking about.

- Answer with facts and supporting documents.

- Make sure that if you have the documents requested and noted in Form 483 that you provide them to the inspector there and then and make a note that you have done so to include it in your response to Form 483.

- Ask for clarification if you do not understand the finding as to which part of the Code of Federal Regulations it refers.

- Have personnel available who may assist in the response to issues raised during the inspection.

- Be polite.

3.17.2   What Is Form 483?

Form 483 is a standard format that the FDA utilizes to provide a written document of the on-site observations of establishment inspections of regulated activities. Form 483 describes any inspectional observations that, in the opinion of the FDA personnel conducting the inspection, represent deviations from applicable statutes and regulations. Since it is the opinion of the inspector, it may be reviewed further by other officers within the FDA. That means that those initial observations may trigger further findings that were not addressed at the exit interview. Therefore, since the observations presented in Form 483 may not always constitute all the findings, the inspector collects copies of all documentation that may support further action (by now you should have an identical set of copies). A published sample of Form 483 is provided in Figure 3.1 for illustrative purposes to allow the reader to understand

DEPARTMENT OF HEALTH AND HUMAN SERVICES	
FOOD AND DRUG ADMINISTRATION	
DISTRICT OFFICE ADDRESS AND PHONE NUMBER 900 Madison Avenue Baltimore, MD 21201 410-962-3396	DATE(S) OF INSPECTION 6/18,19,20,21,28/01
	FEI NUMBER 3003350724
NAME AND TITLE OF INDIVIDUAL TO WHOM REPORT IS ISSUED **TO:** [blank]	
FIRM NAME [blank] Asthma & Allergy Clinic	STREET ADDRESS [blank]
CITY, STATE AND ZIP CODE Baltimore, MD 21224	TYPE OF ESTABLISHMENT INSPECTED Clinical Investigator

DURING AN INSPECTION OF YOUR FIRM, I OBSERVED:

The following observations are related to [blank], entitled, "Mechanisms of Deep [blank]."

1. This sponsor/clinical investigator failed to submit an IND to the FDA prior to conducting this clinical investigation, which involved the administration of [blank] by inhalation to 3 human subjects.

2. The sponsor/clinical investigator failed to report an unanticipated adverse event to the IRB. The first subject in the study,   , was administered [blank] on 4/23/01. She developed a persistent cough from 4/25/01 till 5/3/01. The IRB was not notified of this event.

3. Failure to follow the protocol in that the protocol stated that [blank] would be administered by inhalation, when in fact; [blank] and sodium bicarbonate were actually administered to the second and third subjects.

4. This sponsor/clinical investigator made changes to the approved protocol, dated 9/18/00, without notifying the IRB and without IRB approval, for example:

   a. The sponsor/clinical investigator added sodium bicarbonate to the [blank] to change its pH, for the second and third subjects, without notifying and obtaining approval from the IRB. There were no records available for review to determine how much sodium bicarbonate was added.

   b. The protocol approved by the IRB, dated 9/18/00, stated that the "subjects will be premedicated with either [blank], or its vehicle (normal saline), by inhalation." The clinical investigator administered 4.5% hyperosmolar saline instead of the normal saline.

5. Failure to obtain effective informed consents from subjects, in that the sponsor/clinical investigator failed to disclose that [blank] on administration of [blank] was an experimental use of the drug.

SEE REVERSE OF THIS PAGE	EMPLOYEE(S) SIGNATURE	EMPLOYEE(S) NAME AND TITLE (Print or Type)	DATE ISSUED 6/28/01

Figure 3.1   FDA Form 483: edition obsolete. Inspectional Observations (8/00). Previous

the form. In the illustrative example, the reader can observe that the letter has only five main serious findings to which the investigator has to respond satisfactorily at that point.

3.17.3 Responding to a Form 483

The clinical investigator may respond to some of Form 483 observations verbally during the exit interview. **Nevertheless, a written response is usually expected after the inspection: verbal responses are hard to document.** A comprehensive and timely written response is important to generate a document trail supporting the resolution of any noncompliance issue. The response to Form 483 should be directed to the FDA District Office listed in the upper left-hand corner of Form 483 (see Figure 3.1). However, as noted, Form 483 may not be a complete summary of the findings. After the inspector leaves the investigator site, he/she will inform the district office of the results of the inspection. The inspector will write the internal report to the district office and the investigator will not have access to it. Depending on the seriousness of the violations, the report may be in abbreviated format or full format.

For illustrative purposes, the abbreviated internal format report will be discussed to allow the reader to understand the following steps after a response to the initial inspectional findings is written.

The FDA inspector will have to include the following items in his/her internal inspection report:

1. *Reason for Inspection*

    (a) Identify the headquarter unit that initiated and/or issued the assignment.

    (b) State the purpose of the inspection (premarket approval inspection, compliance inspection, other).

2. *What Was Covered.* Identify the clinical study, protocol number, sponsor, NDA/PMA/PLA/ANDA, and so on (the investigator will know this part since it will correspond to all the documents requested during the inspection).

3. *Location of the Study.* Here the address will be included according to the information provided in Form 1572 and the actual location.

4. *Administrative Procedures*

    (a) The inspector will report the name, title, and authority of the person to whom credentials were shown and FDA Form 482—Notice of Inspection was issued. That person will be the one who the investigator assigned to greet and to assist the inspector during the inspection.

    (b) The inspector will also report the names of all the persons interviewed during the inspection together with their functions and authority.

    (c) The inspector must include the name of the FDA inspector who accompanied him/her during inspection.

    (d) The inspector must report on who provided relevant information to the findings (mainly the coordinator or investigator).

5. The identification of the IRB is important since it may prompt a concurrent or subsequent inspection to the IRB, depending on the findings at the site.

6. The inspector must refer to prior inspectional history, if any, to substantiate further findings and/or corrective actions.

7. *Individual Responsibilities*

   (a) The inspector will identify study personnel and summarize their responsibilities relative to the clinical study. All personnel identified in the organizational chart of the site will be included according to their participation in the study.

   (b) Statement about who obtained informed consent and how it was obtained.

   (c) Identify by whom the trial was monitored and when. Here, if the study was monitored by a third party as a CRO, it has to be identified and, depending on the findings, the CRO may be inspected further.

8. *Inspectional Findings.* In this part the inspector will summarize all violative findings, which the district office will analyze in detail and for which the district office will issue a warning letter if the response to Form 483 was not satisfactory. These inspectional findings will contain the following:

   (a) A statement about comparison of data recorded on the case report forms or tables supplied by the center with the clinical investigator's source documents. (Note that data should be identical and no changes or alterations should be found.)

   (b) Description of which records were covered: that is, patient charts, hospital records, lab slips, and so on (therefore, they must be available and ready for inspection).

   (c) Number of files and case report forms reviewed out of the total study population. (Here the inspector will describe if, having started from a discrete sample, he/she had to broaden when findings were serious.)

   (d) A statement that test article accountability records were or were not sufficient.

   (e) A discussion of Form 483 observations, making reference to the exhibits/documentation collected. (This is the main reason the investigator must retain a copy of all documentation copied by the inspector.)

   (f) The inspector must state whether there was evidence of underreporting of adverse experiences/events. (As an investigator, you should take note that there will be issues regarding your medical opinion of what constitutes an adverse event and its seriousness and severity. The best thing to do in this case is to document in detail all adverse events or issues that may bring an observation during an inspection.)

   (g) A statement about protocol adherence.

9. *Discussion with Management.* Here the inspector must summarize the discussion of the inspectional observations during the exit interview, with the investigator or representative at the site. That discussion will include:

(a) Form 483 observations and non-Form 483 observations.(When non-Form 483 observations are discussed, this means that ancillary aspects will be included that the investigator will not be aware of, such as how approachable the personnel were, or how available the records were, or the general attitudes of the personnel or any other item that may help the center to make a stronger case.)

(b) Discussion of the clinical investigator's response to observations. (The clinical investigator should be prepared with facts to dialog with the inspectors and should be knowledgeable of the requirements and GCP. The investigator must demonstrate that he/she was thoroughly involved with the study and the status of each patient, or had a supervised delegate who did so.)

10. *Sample Collection.* Routine collection of samples from clinical investigators is not normally done. However, if there is a reason that prompted the inspector to suspect the investigational product, such as color, size, shape, dosage form, or route of administration, and the placebo or control, the inspector will collect one package of each for further testing by the FDA.

Now the investigator knows from the contents of this report what the inspector is looking for and what documentation has to be provided to allow the inspector to complete a report. The clinical investigator should know that if information is not provided on the items requested in a report, it could be reported as not provided or not available and this would constitute a violation of the Code of Federal Regulations.

3.17.4 The Follow-up

After the inspection is completed, and the internal inspection report is written, the inspector submits the report, Form 483, and the supporting documents to the assigned center, and your inspectional observations will be dealt with further by the center. You may not be contacted any more by the inspector or write to him/her regarding your inspection since his/her job is done. From now on, you will be dealing with the assigned officer at the regional center who will identify him/herself in further communications to you.

There are many forms of communications that the FDA may utilize to proceed further with your case; however, the main way would be in the form of a "Warning Letter."

3.17.5 Warning Letter

Warning letters are issued by the corresponding FDA district office after an inspection where a Form 483 was issued and the clinical investigator's response to Form 483 was not satisfactory to address the main issues. The warning letter process intends to prompt the investigator (or stakeholder) to take actions that are deemed satisfactory to the regulator to guarantee that violations do not occur in the future.

The redaction of a warning letter may correspond to a typical format as follows:

Between the dates of [blank] and [blank], [name of the inspector(s) – District office], representing the Food and Drug Administration (FDA), conducted an investigation and met with you to review your conduct of a clinical investigation of the following clinical study (ies) [blank] sponsored by [blank].

This inspection is a part of the FDA's Bioresearch Monitoring Program, which includes inspections designed to evaluate the conduct of research and to ensure that the rights, safety, and welfare of the human subjects of the study have been protected. From our review of the establishment inspection report, the documents submitted with that report, and your [date] written response to FDA Form 483, we conclude that you did not adhere to the applicable statutory requirements and FDA regulations governing the conduct of clinical investigations and the protection of human subjects. We wish to emphasize the following...

This part of the warning letter is standard to any party inspected and intends to introduce and justify the reason for the warning.

The next part of the warning letter enumerates in detail the violations with respect of the Code of Federal Regulations (CFR) and the findings pinpointing the detail that prompted the observation. In every case the letter will include verbatim what is expected from the investigator according to the requirements in the respective part of the CFR. The detail of the particular findings in the clinical investigator's warning letter is discussed in the section entitled Analysis of Warning Letters to Clinical Investigators."

The ending of the warning letter also corresponds to a typical format as follows:

This letter is not intended to be an all-inclusive list of deficiencies with your clinical study of an investigational drug. It is your responsibility to ensure adherence to each requirement of the law and relevant FDA regulations. You must address these deficiencies and establish procedures to ensure that any on-going or future studies will be in compliance with FDA regulations.

Within fifteen (15) working days of your receipt of this letter, you must notify this office in writing of the actions you have taken or will be taking to prevent similar violations in the future. In your written response, you have acknowledged the regulatory violations, however, you have failed to provide us with adequate assurances or corrective measures to prevent similar violations from recurring in the future. Failure to adequately and promptly explain the violations noted above may result in regulatory action without further notice.

If you have any questions, please contact [district office chief]. Your written response and any pertinent documentation should be addressed to: [blank]

As you can observe, the letter is written by an officer of the assigned district; however, you will be responding to the district office chief responsible for the branch. The clinical investigator has to understand that a team was assigned to deal with the violations and that he/she will be addressing members of the team as requested. (Note that in Canada, on the contrary, when a Health Canada inspector conducts a GCP inspection, he/she is the one to be contacted until all issues are resolved.)

Analyzing sentence by sentence the closing of the warning letter, we can observe the following:

"This letter is not intended to be an all-inclusive list of deficiencies with your clinical study of an investigational drug"

This means that you cannot rest assured that the FDA found all of your deficiencies, but it has identified you as a clinical investigator who has not complied with requirements and regulations. Simply stated, there may be more violations. Now, how do you know if there are more issues that were not uncovered by the FDA but that may hinder a market application, for example? It is the duty of the sponsor (in the case of a pharmaceutical, medical device, or biologic company) to provide for quality assurance to determine compliance. If the investigator is also the sponsor, then the investigator should have procedures to determine adherence to regulatory requirements, GCP, and the protocol. The latter is harder to achieve, since most of the investigator-initiated studies do not have the necessary expertise for QA audits. Therefore, it is highly recommended that investigator-initiated studies are audited by a third party expert to give the site the quality assurance necessary to determine compliance.

"It is your responsibility to ensure adherence to each requirement of the law and relevant FDA regulations."

Obviously, here the regulator underlines that you, the clinical investigator, signed Form 1572 or assumed the responsibilities of an investigator, and bear that responsibility.

"You must address these deficiencies and establish procedures to ensure that any on-going or future studies will be in compliance with FDA regulations."

Here is the clue; this is what the FDA wants from you. In your response to the warning letter (or to Form 483) the FDA wants you to establish procedures to ensure that any on-going or future studies will be in compliance with FDA regulations, and the issue is that you must convince the FDA that you can implement them as well as train your personnel in following those procedures.

If you read this book from the beginning, there are no established GCP requirements for the clinical investigator to implement standard operating procedures or have a quality assurance program since protocol adherence is the key to compliance. However, once an inspection determines that you as a clinical investigator "failed" to adhere, the only assurance that the regulator can have that violations will not happen in the future is to request procedures.

Remember that procedures alone will not help your site become more compliant, but adequate training in regulatory requirements and a quality assurance process will.

Training and quality assurance imply a cost that has to be included in the cost to run clinical trials at the site.

Another paragraph indicates the following:

Within fifteen (15) working days of your receipt of this letter, you must notify this office in writing of the actions you have taken or will be taking to prevent similar violations in the future. In your written response, you have acknowledged the regulatory violations, however, you have failed to provide us with adequate assurances or corrective measures to prevent similar violations from recurring in the future.

The FDA wants details of all the procedures that you plan to implement, including copies of the written procedures, as well as a training program for your personnel on those procedures, and timelines for implementation. Fifteen days may be too short to put together a procedure manual, but the clinical investigator must respond with all the plans to date and how they are going to be implemented. Future correspondence should include a copy of all the required procedures.

"Failure to adequately and promptly explain the violations noted above may result in regulatory action without further notice."

Basically, the clinical investigator is not provided with options; therefore, a qualified response must be issued to conclude the issue. The process of responding to the regulator requests may take longer than expected. But what if the responses do not satisfy the regulator by providing assurance that the violations will not occur in the future? The regulator may initiate regulatory actions, as indicated in the following sections, against the investigator until he/she is convinced that the site will not fail to adhere to requirements, the investigator may even not be allowed to participate in clinical trials.

3.17.6 Regulatory Actions Against Clinical Investigators

Clinical investigators are selected by the sponsors according a certain criteria and their willingness to comply with Section 50 "Protection of Human Subjects" and Section 56 "Institutional Review Boards" of 21 CFR, or they may initiate a clinical study by themselves (investigator-initiated clinical trial) but they also must comply with a sponsor's responsibilities. Additionally, once the investigator signs Form 1572, he/she assumes the responsibilities of an investigator and has to comply with Subpart D 21 CFR 312.50 to 21 CFR 312.58 as well as good clinical practices, and the clinical trial protocol.

The investigator can be inspected by the FDA at any time. If an inspection demonstrates with enough evidence serious violations (purposely or unintentionally) of the above-mentioned requirements, or the investigator has submitted false or misleading information to the FDA, after warning letters, a disqualification procedure could be initiated.

Notice of Initiation of Disqualification Proceeding and Opportunity to Explain (NIDPOE) (312.70) This letter is issued to a clinical investigator who failed to respond appropriately to the requests of the FDA or submitted purposely false or misleading information. A NIDPOE letter is a serious matter and the clinical investigator should respond accordingly. That letter provides the investigator with written notice of the matter and offers the investigator an opportunity to explain the matter in writing, or, at the option of the investigator, in an informal conference. NIDPOE letters are published in the FDA website once they are issued. A total of six NIDPOE letters were issued in 2008; the same number were issued in 2007.

The disqualification procedure may involve the following:

1. *The Informal Conference.* In this conference the investigator is provided with an opportunity to explain verbally instead of writing a letter. If an informal conference is held, the investigator may also bring an attorney.

2. *Opportunity for a Regulatory Hearing.* If, after hearing in the informal conference the investigator's explanation, the center still believes that the investigator's actions meet the threshold for disqualification, the center must offer the investigator an opportunity for a regulatory hearing, whose procedures are governed by 21 CFR Part 16 (21 CFR 312.70). The investigator may enter into a consent agreement at any time or may request a hearing. At a regulatory hearing, the investigator may offer the testimony of witnesses, documentary evidence, and supporting briefs.

3. *Disqualification.* After the hearing, the presiding officer issues a report or decision on whether the investigator has repeatedly or deliberately violated the regulations and should be disqualified. The report is forwarded to the Commissioner, who then issues a Commissioner's Decision on Disqualification (21 CFR Part 16). The investigator may appeal the Commissioner's decision in federal court. A disqualification proceeding generally takes many months or years to complete.

What is a Disqualification of an Investigator?   The disqualification means that the investigator is completely banned to participate in a clinical trial under any conditions, and the disqualified or "totally restricted" clinical investigator is not eligible to receive investigational drugs, biologics, or devices. Additionally, the investigator will be immediately added to the disqualified/restricted/restrictions removed/assurances list for.[2]

If criminal actions are suspected, the FDA may initiate a civil or criminal enforcement action in federal court. Such actions can take several months and frequently years to complete.

What is the Consent Agreement?   The clinical investigator can apply for a consent agreement at any time. The FDA, in some instances, may allow clinical investigators to enter into "restricted agreements" when the agency believes that lesser sanctions than disqualification would be adequate to protect the public health. The decision to offer a "restricted agreement" is within the discretion of the FDA. Clinical investigators on this list[3] may still be eligible to receive investigational products, provided they conduct regulated studies in accordance with the restrictions specified in their agreement with the FDA and all applicable regulatory requirements. Those conditions may be temporary until the investigator provides adequate assurances with respect to future compliance with requirements applicable to the use of investigational drugs and biologics.

3.17.7   The Clinical Hold

A clinical hold is an order by the FDA that immediately suspends or imposes restrictions on an ongoing or proposed clinical study (21 CFR 312.42). The suspension may affect (1) only the site for an investigator who was identified being in violation of the Code of Federal Regulations, or (2) the entire study.

---

[2]http://www.fda.gov/ICECI/EnforcementActions/DisqualifiedRestrictedAssuranceList/ucm131681.htm

[3]http://www.fda.gov/ICECI/EnforcementActions/DisqualifiedRestrictedAssuranceList/ucm131684.htm

The clinical hold may be applied before or after an enforcement action has been initiated against the investigator. The timing will depend on the type of misconduct detected and the risk to the human subjects exposed to the investigational product that are under the care of the investigator. Nevertheless, the FDA will, unless patients are exposed to immediate and serious risk, attempt to discuss and satisfactorily resolve the matter with the sponsor before issuing the clinical hold order [21 CFR 312.42(c)]. If possible, as in all cases where a clinical hold is considered, the FDA will contact the sponsor and attempt to resolve the matter in a way that adequately protects study subjects before imposing a clinical hold, following the time frames described in companion guidances and regulations [e.g., *Guidance with Industry: Formal Meetings with Sponsors and Applicants for PDUFA Products* and 21 CFR 312.42(e) respectively]. In those cases where an inspection appears necessary to resolve issues, the FDA will make every effort to ensure that the inspections are completed in a timely manner.

Issue of the Clinical Hold   A clinical hold is an order issued by the FDA to the sponsor to delay a proposed clinical investigation or to suspend an ongoing investigation. The contact will initially be by telephone, followed by a written document.

Scope of the Clinical Hold   The clinical hold order may apply to one or more of the investigations covered by an IND. This means that the study may continue for some sites, but be suspended for other sites.

Meaning of the Clinical Hold   When a proposed study (one that has not started yet) is placed on clinical hold, subjects may not be given the investigational drug.

When an ongoing study is placed on clinical hold, no new subjects may be recruited to the study and placed on the investigational drug; patients already in the study should be taken off therapy involving the investigational drug unless specifically permitted to remain in therapy by the FDA in the interest of patient safety.

Extent of the Clinical Hold   A clinical hold may be complete or partial. Delay or suspension of all clinical work under an IND is considered a complete clinical hold. Delay or suspension of only part of the clinical work under an IND is considered a partial clinical hold. A partial clinical hold could, for example, be imposed to delay or suspend one of several protocols in an IND, a part of a protocol, or a specific study site in a multisite investigation.

The FDA's regulation authorizing clinical holds on studies of drugs and biological products sets forth grounds for imposing a hold. Those grounds vary depending on the nature of the study. For all types of studies, however, the FDA may impose a clinical hold if it finds that "human subjects are or would be exposed to an unreasonable and significant risk of illness or injury" [21 CFR 312.42(b)(1)(i), (b)(2)(i), (b)(3)(i)(A), (b)(3)(ii)(E)(2), (b)(4)(i), (b)(5)(i), (b)(6)(i)].

From the point of view of a sponsor of a clinical investigation, a clinical hold, if it is due to other reasons than significant risk to humans, is a matter that could jeopardize the entire development, delaying at a point where it becomes unreasonable to continue with the plan (e.g., patent expiration).

Lift of the Clinical Hold   The FDA will lift a clinical hold imposed to protect subjects from investigator misconduct when the grounds for the hold no longer apply (the grounds of the hold are removed).The sponsor of the affected study may, while the clinical hold is in place, present evidence to the FDA to show that it has taken steps to protect study subjects (e.g., by replacing the investigator who is charged with the misconduct or, in the case of a sponsor–investigator, by submitting a monitoring plan). If the FDA concludes, based on this evidence, that the study subjects are no longer exposed to an unreasonable and significant risk of illness or injury, the hold will be lifted. In all instances, if a sponsor of a study that has been placed on clinical hold requests in writing that the clinical hold be removed and responds to the issues identified in the clinical hold order, the FDA will respond in writing to the sponsor within 30 calendar days of receipt of the request [21 CFR 312.42(e)]. The FDA will either remove or maintain the clinical hold and will state the reasons for its decision.

3.17.8   Reinstatement of Disqualified Investigators

An investigator who has been determined to be ineligible to receive investigational drugs may be reinstated[4] as eligible when the Commissioner determines that the investigator has presented adequate assurances that the investigator will employ investigational drugs solely in compliance with the provisions of Part 312, 50 and 56 of the Code of Federal Regulations.

3.17.9   Regulatory Action Against Companies or Persons (Not Investigators): Debarment

Firms or individuals[5] convicted of a felony under federal law for conduct (by a firm) relating to the development or approval, including the process for development or approval, of any abbreviated drug application; or (an individual convicted) for conduct relating to development or approval of any drug product, or otherwise relating to any drug product under the Federal Food, Drug, and Cosmetic Act can be debarred from the activity and will be included in this list. Under the law, a debarred person can't work for a drug firm "in any capacity." According to the U.S. Court of Appeals for the District of Columbia, even a job as a cook in a drug firm's cafeteria would be forbidden because of the opportunity for close contact between the debarred person and the drug firm's management. "All direct employment by a drug company, whether in the board room or the cafeteria or somewhere in between" is forbidden, the court said. Besides direct employment, some jobs for a contractor that provides services to a drug firm are also prohibited. Debarment is a serious measure, but it's not intended to be a punishment. Its intention is to protect the public by ensuring that people with a history of dishonest conduct in the drug approval process will no longer be participants in that process. Although debarment is considered mandatory and permanent, the debarred person/firm could apply for *termination*.

---

[4]http://www.fda.gov/ICECI/EnforcementActions/DisqualifiedRestrictedAssuranceList/ucm131690.htm
[5]http://www.fda.gov/ICECI/EnforcementActions/FDADebarmentList/ucm2005408.htm

CHAPTER 4

ANALYSIS OF WARNING LETTERS

4.1 ANALYSIS OF WARNING LETTERS ISSUED TO CLINICAL INVESTIGATORS AND THE IMPACT ON PRODUCT DEVELOPMENT

This book has already dealt with the standard aspects of the warning letters as to the introductory statements and the closing arguments and requests. In this chapter the focus will be on the findings and the regulatory implications.

Each finding will be discussed as presented in the warning letters available online.

4.1.1 Most Common Findings of Investigator Site Inspections

Findings Relating to Patient Information and Consent Form and Process

(1) You failed to obtain informed consent of the subjects to whom the study drug was administered. (21 CFR § 312.60; 21 CFR § 50.20)

The consent process and the consent form must be in compliance with the above-mentioned requirements. Investigators often misunderstand or underestimate the extent of the applicability of the consent process.

For example, an observation in a warning letter stated the following:

Section x,y of Protocol required that subjects sign the informed consent document (ICD) to indicate they understood the purpose of the study and procedures. The protocol also stated that subjects would be excluded if they could not provide their own consent. The investigation found that a guardian signed the ICD for Subject X on [date]. The sponsor recommended this subject be immediately discontinued from the study for consenting reasons on [date].

This observation demonstrated that the investigator (or consenter) did not understand the extent of the consent process as to who should sign the document and proceeded to enroll a patient who could not sign by him/herself. Although it is allowed to have guardians or legal representatives sign on behalf of a patient (21 CFR 50), that has to be incorporated in the protocol and the consent process and approved by the IRB.

Your response letter dated June 6, 2006 did not address the issue of consent related to Subject X. Your letter did address the issue of informed consent related to Subject Y.

Clinical Trials Audit Preparation: A Guide for Good Clinical Practice (GCP) Inspections, by Vera Mihajlovic-Madzarevic
Copyright © 2010 John Wiley & Sons, Inc.

This subject consented to the open-label phase of the study while hospitalized and suffering periods of delusion. You assert that this subject's consent was valid in part because the subject had been informed of the open-label phase of the trial at the time the subject first consented to trial participation. This assertion is improper. Knowledge of trial phases does not suffice to demonstrate informed consent to those phases. Moreover, a subject can withdraw consent at any time during a study, which underscores the fact that informed consent must be established independently at each trial phase required under the protocol. [21 CFR § 50.25(a)(8)]

The investigator cannot assume that a patient agreeing to one part of a clinical study will consent to another phase. The fact is that the subject MUST comply with all the requirements of the protocol to consent, and one of them was to provide his/her own consent for each phase or else be excluded.

This also underscores how hard it is for a clinical investigator to retain patients in a clinical trial, and how difficult it is to remain compliant with extremely complicated protocols.

(2) You failed to meet the requirements for informed consent, specifically the requirement that information given to the subject or the subject's representative shall be in language understandable to the subject or the representative. (21 CFR 50.20)

Consent forms should be written in a language that the patient or representative can understand. In countries where more than one language or dialect is spoken, the investigator should have consent forms properly translated and approved by institutional review boards. Moreover, once a consent document is written in language other than the official language, the entire form should be written in that language, and the entire document should be consented to at once. For example, a misinterpretation of the requirement may render the following observation:

The study Research Subject Information and Consent Form signed by Subject C dated January 3, 2007 is 12 pages long, with the first eight pages written in the English language and the last four pages written in the Spanish language. There was no documentation that this subject is bilingual in both English and Spanish. The section of the consent with seven questions requiring a "yes" or "no" response, appearing in Spanish language text, **is not** completed. The Research Authorization signed by L on January 3, 2007 consists of the first three pages in English and the signature last page in Spanish. All English language versions of these consent forms dated March 16, 2007 were signed by C however; there is no signature or date relating to the individual discussing the consent. Subject L completed study participation on/or about March 14, 2007.

(3) You failed to obtain informed consent of subjects involved in research in accordance with the provisions of 21 CFR Part 50. (21 CFR 312.601)

For example,

Subject X signed a sub-study consent document, but did not sign an informed consent document for participation in the main study.

Here we are again facing the problem of very complex studies where protocols may have several parts that can be consented individually. The investigator should train personnel extensively to ensure that they are aware of all parts of the consent process and do not handle the wrong form (either a draft or a part that does not correspond).

Four of 23 subjects [redacted] had protocol-specified baseline laboratory blood samples drawn prior to signing and dating the informed consent document.

or

Subject 2006 had study assessments and procedures performed during the screening visit on February 2, 2007; however, the subject did not sign the informed consent form approved by the Institutional Review Board (IRB) until May 18, 2007.

This issue has to do with the misconception that until investigational product is dispensed, consent need not be obtained. That is **absolutely wrong**.

Consent should be obtained prior to submitting the patient to any trial related procedure, including a trial-related questionnaire or collecting subject's data for a clinical trial.

Remember that during a baseline period, the patient is going to provide personal information and samples or participate in tests that otherwise would not be necessary for his/her condition and they pose a risk.

The IRB approved informed consent document required documentation of the actual time in which legally effective informed consent of the subject was obtained. There was no documentation of the actual time in which subjects [redacted] signed and dated the consent forms. In addition, we were unable to verify that these subjects signed and dated the informed consent forms prior to any protocol specified procedures being conducted on them.

It is very common that when consent is signed on the same day that the first clinical trial-related activity is initiated, that the time of consent is included with the date. In this case, it was a requirement of the IRB; however, the investigator failed to record the time. This finding may have serious implications since it may presuppose that a patient is included for baseline and eligibility testing and, if eligible, consented after the fact. That goes also against the Declaration of Helsinki.

In your September 18, 2007 written response, you noted that in all cases the subject had verbally consented prior to any study procedures being performed. Verbal consent, however, is inadequate. The exceptions in 21 CFR 50.23 and 21 CFR 50.24 to the informed consent requirements, as well as the exception in 21 CFR 56.109(c) to use of the written consent form approved by the IRB, did not apply to the conduct of this study.

First, GCP and the FDA require that written consent be obtained. Second, verbal consent may be allowed in exceptional circumstances when the IRBs approve it. This was not the case. It is extremely important that all investigators understand that clinical research is not medical practice and that strict adherence to regulations is required to guarantee subject's rights and safety.

One of the subjects enrolled in the study signed the consent form for the incorrect study. Specifically, Subject [redacted] signed the 1/19/01 version of the consent form on

8/12/03, which was dated as approved by the IRB on 3/20/01, for the original clinical study. Enrollment for the original study was completed in February 2002, and additional subjects should have been enrolled into the [redacted] with a new informed consent form dated 3/10/03. The old consent form contained the incorrect address for the IRB, and differed in study purpose, the sponsor name, and patient confidentiality information.

or

Subject 2005 had study assessments and procedures performed for protocol Y on January 18, 2007 at the screening visit; however, the subject signed a consent form for another study, protocol X and did not sign the consent form for participation in protocol Y until March 6, 2007.

Using the wrong consent form is a serious matter and indicates that the clinical trial personnel are not adequately trained in the clinical trial and did not understand the implications of having a proper consent process. If thorough discussion of the clinical trial procedures with the patient had taken place, the error would have been identified and proper consent provided. Also, clinical trial sites running several studies for different sponsors should have appropriate resources to handle all documentation properly. Signing the wrong form means that the patient did not consent for the study and therefore was enrolled without consent. This is a serious violation.

Subject [redacted] had the [redacted] on 7/11/03, but the consent was not signed until 7/21/03. A handwritten note on the consent form states, "I was informed about study and the risk—did not sign consent 6-26-03," but the note is not signed or dated by the study subject. In addition, there was nothing in the subject's clinic record to confirm that she verbally consented prior to the [redacted]. Where consent is obtained orally, it must be documented on an IRB-approved short form consent document in accordance with 21 CFR 50.27(b)(2).

or

During the FDA inspection you were not able to provide signed informed consent documents for subject XX. You told the FDA investigator that this subject signed an informed consent document, but you could not locate the document. Inspection revealed that the caregiver could not recall an informed consent document being signed.

This is a clear example of a site finding out that either it failed to obtain consent before clinical trial procedures are initiated or lost the signed form and no reference in the patient file is done. In that case, the patient should have been discontinued and the reason should be stated as "consent not properly obtained."

None of the subjects dated the Informed Consent Document per your own admission at the time of the inspection, when you stated that you dated the Informed Consent Documents of all participating subjects.

It is very critical that when subjects are enrolled in a study and sign the patient information and consent form that they use their own pen and sign and date it themselves. It is not acceptable that the site stamps or types the dates or the coordinator includes the dates. There must be evidence that the subject acknowledged the time of signature.

There is no documentation available to indicate that a copy of the signed and dated Informed Consent Document was provided to each subject. This was confirmed by your own admission to the FDA Field Investigator at the time of the inspection that you did not provide the subjects a copy of the signed Informed Consent Document.

21 CFR 50.57(a) establishes that a copy of the written consent be provided to the patient at the time of the signature on the consent form. The copy should not be a photocopied consent, but another original for the patient to take home and have available at any time for reference. It is important that the copy be provided immediately because the description of the study is in there as well as contact numbers in case the patient has any question or issue and a description of the patient's rights and responsibilities.

You obtained informed consent from some subjects using consent form versions for Study 1 that were not approved by the Institutional Review Board (IRB). Informed consent from the subject is not legally effective if the form that is signed has not been approved by the IRB or if the consent form describes the wrong procedures.... Signed a revised informed consent form (3/27/00) before it was approved by the IRB on 4/4/00....

The investigator cannot use a revised or amended consent form before it is approved by the IRB. Any information provided to the patient must be previously approved by the IRB.

(4) Legally effective informed consent was not obtained from a subject or the subject's legally authorized representative. (21 CFR 812.100, 50.20, 50.23, and 50.27)

This is a worst case scenario. The patient may not have signed an IRB approved consent form or consent at all before initiating a study-related activity/procedure.

Our investigation found that for 30 of the 34 subjects enrolled, informed consent was not obtained or documented by the use of a written consent form approved by the IRB and signed and dated by the subject or the subject's legally authorized representative at the time of consent.

Findings Relating to Investigator's Supervision of the Clinical Trial

(a) Failure to personally conduct or adequately supervise the above-referenced clinical trial. (21 CFR 312.60)

The clinical trial investigator, by signing Form 1572, assumes the responsibility of personally conducting the study or supervising the personnel conducting the study. It is observed in many cases that there is not even an arm's length relationship between the principal investigator and the clinical trial personnel. The observation goes further:

You specifically agreed to personally conduct the clinical study or to supervise those aspects of the study that you did not personally conduct....While you may delegate certain study tasks to individuals qualified to perform them, as a clinical investigator you may not delegate your general responsibilities. Our investigation indicates that your supervision of personnel to whom you delegated study tasks was not adequate to ensure that the clinical trial was conducted according to the signed investigator statement, the investigational plan, and applicable regulations, and in a manner that protects the rights, safety, and welfare of human subjects. . . . Our investigation indicates that you had little personal involvement in the conduct of the study beyond referring patients from your practice for enrollment in the study, conducting physical examinations, and reviewing screening ECGs, and that you failed to adequately supervise individuals who performed study tasks.

The investigator should organize the clinical trial site with an established control process through standard operating procedures, where points of personal supervision exist and documents are generated to prove a personal involvement for all established procedures in the protocol or else the following may happen:

Although the protocol (section 5.5.1) required that the investigator review all available assessments at the screening/baseline visit (e.g., vital signs, current medications, concomitant medical conditions, inclusion/exclusion criteria) to ensure subject eligibility for the study, statements made by you and Ms. C to the FDA investigator, indicate that your study coordinator, Ms. L screened and enrolled study subjects.

or worse still

It is not clear if Ms. L was qualified to perform the duties that were delegated to her. . . your study coordinator enrolled multiple subjects who were not eligible for inclusion in the study (met exclusion criteria).

All these observations render the following logical conclusion:

Your lack of supervision and personal involvement, and inappropriate delegation of study tasks, resulted in failure to protect the rights, safety, and welfare of study subjects, failure to adhere to the study protocol, failure to maintain adequate and accurate study records, and failure to promptly report serious adverse events to the sponsor and IRB.

The point here is that if an investigator considers that personal involvement or supervision is not possible due to other previously agreed activities, he/she cannot agree to "host" a site and have third parties running the study without proper supervision. The bottom line is that a principal investigator is being engaged by the sponsor to provide his/her expertise to the assessment of safety and efficacy of an investigational product. If that principal investigator cannot assume the responsibility of supervision of patients, the spirit of having a principal investigator is contradicted. Another source of misunderstanding is that the investigator may consider the coordinator/ research assistant qualified by experience to perform certain duties, such as checking and deciding on the eligibility of patients to be enrolled in the study. It is important to understand that qualification in cases where decisions are made on patient's care, means qualification by education and experience, such as being a medical professional or registered nurse, if applicable. The determination of eligibility for a clinical trial, ergo investigational medical treatment, is the responsibility of a qualified medical investigator for the reason that when the investigator decides to include a patient in a study, it is because he/she considers it in the best interest of the patient from the medical point of view. Therefore, although the coordinator may know exactly which criteria a patient has to fulfill to be entered in a study, the final decision has to be made by the qualified investigator *and documented*. If the coordinator is medically qualified to perform such assessment, then a proper written process of delegation of that responsibility should be available, together with the documentation to justify that qualification.

Another clear example is the following:

> For [NN] protocol, you delegated the performance of protocol-specified clinical evaluations (e.g., physical examinations, and evaluation of signs and symptoms relating to a DVT or pulmonary embolism) to [XX]. According to the Site Personnel Delegation Log, [XX] was assigned a role of data entry for CRFs. During the inspection, Mr. [XX] indicated that he was not trained or qualified to perform physical examinations, and other required assessments. For example, . . . for Subject [YY] the Day 65 physical examination and DVT/PE assessment was performed by [XX] during a visit date of March 19, 2007, while you were in England.

This evidence speaks for itself. Critical responsibilities were directly or indirectly delegated to an unqualified individual. For more information, please review the FDA Guidance for Industry, Investigator Responsibilities—Protecting the Rights, Safety, and Welfare of Study Subjects issued October 2009.

Findings Relating to Protocol Adherence

(1) You failed to conduct the clinical investigations according to the investigational plans. (21 CFR 312.60)

Together with the findings noted earlier, lack of protocol adherence is a common finding where principal investigators do not follow strictly the protocol requirements; for example,

> Of nine subjects randomized in Protocol three subjects met exclusionary criteria, but were not excluded from the study.

Regarding this observation, we can establish several reasons why the wrong patient was included because the inclusion/exclusion criteria were not followed. The investigator may assume that, in his/her medical opinion, the patient's condition is acceptable; and so a patient otherwise not eligible for study enrollment is enrolled. Although this appears to be reasonable for the investigator, the issue is that, in global or multicenter studies, to maintain general criteria for enrollment it is key to select patients who would further be eligible for efficacy and safety analysis according to preestablished protocol requirements. If noneligible patients are enrolled, the assessments become impossible, since new variables are introduced that were not part of the protocol. Moreover, exclusion criteria mostly take into account serious underlying conditions or concomitant medications that may fatally interact with the study medication, or other factors that may endanger the safety of the patient and thus considerably increase the risk to participate in a study. Therefore, the investigator should always consider, apart from his/her medical opinion on the eligibility of a patient, the safety concerns of the exclusion criteria, which were thoroughly examined and decided on in the protocol design.

Another example of misunderstanding between clinical trial criteria and medical practice is as follows:

> Protocol [XX] prohibited the use of pneumatic compression devices. Records for 5 of 62 subjects documented that they received intermittent foot pneumatic compression during

hospitalization following total knee replacement: [XX] and [XX]. . . . Your response letter dated May 18, 2007 states that the use of intermittent pneumatic foot compression therapy has been a standard of care for the majority of patients at the [XX] Medical Center, and that the personnel continued using this device with the patients enrolled in these studies. DSI considers your response to be unacceptable. The protocol specifically prohibited the use of intermittent pneumatic compression devices. Furthermore, our investigation found an email exchange of September 26, 2006, between [XX] Senior Medical Research Associate, [XX], and Office Manager [XX] specifically stating that use of planned intermittent pneumatic compression during active treatment period was an exclusion criteria.

This issue happens very commonly when the investigator in his/her medical opinion considers that a standard of care cannot be construed as an exclusion. Clinical trials, using investigational medical therapies, must follow strict criteria to control all analyzable parameters.

The following will focus on the *details* in data collection and protocol adherence.

For the [XX] study, the Screening (Day 0) chemistry lab test for Subject [XX] was collected on December 13, 2006. These lab results documented, among other things, a Lactate Dehydrogenase (LDH) value of 1612 U/L (reference range 100–220 U/L), stamped as "not clinically significant." This entry did not contain dates or signatures of the responsible person. The associated "screening" hematology report contained your signature and was dated January 5, 2007, approximately three weeks after this subject's hip replacement surgery on December 19, 2006. No documentation was found explaining the determination that the LDH value was "not clinically significant."

Although the investigator may know the answer for considering out of range lab values as "not clinically significant," that has to be made evident in writing on the lab report or the patient file in a chronological manner. Again, clinical trials collect *all* information regarding safety of a patient, and this is key to safety.

Your response dated May 18, 2007, states that you chose not to require repeat testing because blood work would be performed prior to the subject's surgery as part of the pre-operative hospital procedure. You also noted that it appeared that the initial blood sample was unreliable based on the NSA potassium results, and that chronic or acute tissue damage would have been noted in the subject if the initial LDH value was accurate. You also state that blood collection was performed on the day after surgery, and that the lab values were within normal range. This response is unacceptable. An LDH value of 1612 U/L is clearly out of range, and clinic records should document why you considered this as "not clinically significant." Furthermore, you did not explain why you reviewed the screening chemistry lab results on January 5, 2007, almost three weeks after the subject's surgery.

Although the investigator's decision to continue the patient in the study follows perhaps medical practice criteria, it does not follow clinical trial requirements to document all decisions that may affect patient safety. The inspector requires documentation to support the investigator's decision. Also, inconsistencies in the dates when documents are actually reviewed and signed have to be clarified properly. Many times, an investigator reviews all data and makes a decision on the spot; then, after a while, when completing the CRFs, the investigator signs all supporting documents. That should not be the case.

Here is a clear example of a he said/she said case:

The [XX] Protocol required that blood samples be drawn twice on Day 6, to measure coagulation parameters. The protocol specified the times for these blood draws as shortly before intake of the tablet (at trough) and 2–4 hours after intake of tablet (at peak). For Subject [XX], for the Day 6 sample, the drug administration records document that study drug was administered at 21:21 on February 19, 2007. The post-dose blood collection record documents a time of 22:30, or slightly more than 1 hour later. For Subject [XX] drug administration records document that study drug was administered at 10:19 AM on October 30, 2006, and the blood collection records document a time of 16:00, or almost 8 hours later. ....We acknowledge in your letter dated May 18, 2007, you state that the times entered by the nurse were erroneous, and that the Study Coordinator was present during the period of drug administration and firmly recalls the sample collection times as being done within the timeframes specified by the protocol. DSI considers this response to be inadequate because you provided no documentation to support your contention.

When the investigator responds to an observation as serious as this one, supporting documentation is imperative. Unless the investigator has documentary evidence, any assertion will be considered groundless and therefore refutable (he said/ she said).

Protocol version #2, amendment #2 (dated December 8, 2000) [hereinafter "the protocol"] further clarified this inclusion criterion noting that if the sputum sample at enrollment had <25 WBC/lpf, obtaining another sputum sample that demonstrated >25 WBC/Ipf would be acceptable, provided that the patient has received no more than 48 hrs of study medications at the time the second sputum sample was collected. Subjects [XX] and [XX] were enrolled in the study even though their sputum samples did not have the protocol required inclusion criterion of >25 WBC/lpf. ...

The protocol specified that within 48 hrs prior to enrollment, the subject must provide a purulent or muco-purulent sputum by deep expectoration for gram stain, culture, and susceptibility testing. Subject [XX] was unable to produce the protocol required sputum specimen for enrollment; however you still dispensed study medication to this subject. ...

In your September 18, 2007, written response, you noted that patients coming into the office with an acute infection need to be treated quickly. You further stated that study participants had to be screened, enrolled and randomized in a manner that is typically much faster than for other types of non-infectious disease clinical trials; hence there was no in-depth review of screening with all lab and x-ray data in hand before randomization. This answer is inadequate. FDA regulations require that clinical investigators enrolling subjects into FDA regulated clinical studies follow the investigational plan to help ensure the reliability of data collected during the study and that the rights, safety and welfare of research participants are protected.

Clinical trial investigators have to enroll a certain number of patients in a clinical trial in a limited time frame. Finding patients who fulfill all the criteria is sometimes extremely difficult. In the case of acute infections, although the protocol seems to establish a wait period to determine eligibility, for this investigator standard of care could have meant treating the patient immediately (even with the investigational product). This assumption is wrong and the investigator should have discussed the issue with the sponsor of the study to make it clear that some preestablished time frames for the clinical trial may endanger the welfare of patients. However, as it stands, the protocol should have been followed.

Another example of this is the following:

> The protocol excluded potential subjects who were taking Aleve (naproxen) medication one (1) month prior to the screening visit. The Medical Information Sheet for subject XX at screening documents that the subject was currently taking Aleve; however, the subject was randomized in violation of the protocol.

As we can observe from detailed protocol adherence findings, the lack of in-depth training of medical investigators in clinical trial processes and procedures may render misinterpretations that, a posteriori, are observed as either deviations or violations to the protocol.

(a) You failed to protect the rights, safety, and welfare of subjects under your care. (21 CFR 312.60)

Here is an example:

> Despite the importance for subject safety of monitoring CPK levels, and the protocol's explicit requirements to do so, you did not obtain all required CPK levels or other required laboratory results for any subject you enrolled. . . .
>
> In addition, the protocol provided detailed instructions about what to do if subjects experienced elevated CPK levels. . . .If CPK levels exceed the upper limit of normal by twofold at any time of the trial, the central laboratory will automatically evaluate CPK isoenzymes to determine if the elevated fraction is M/M. Venous blood samples will then be obtained on a daily basis and sent to the central laboratory for CPK monitoring (i.e., CPK will be determined each day, with other serum chemistries determined every other day). If CPK levels subsequently decline to within the normal range, then venous blood samples should be obtained according to the original schedule. If CPK levels exceed [redacted] U/mL, the unblinded investigator will call the medical monitor. A decision to discontinue or continue the subject will be jointly made and will be based on the risk/benefit of continued therapy for the subject. If the subject continues in the trial and CPK levels increase another twofold, the subject must be withdrawn from the study and CPK isoenzymes, serum myoglobin, and urinary myoglobin will be evaluated at the termination visit.

This is a serious finding where the clinical investigator did not adhere to the protocol requirements of lab testing and by doing so endangered the lives of the patients by continuing treatment and not excluding patients as per protocol.

Findings Relating to Records in Clinical Trials

(1) You failed to maintain adequate and accurate case histories that record all observations and other data pertinent to the investigation on each individual. [21 CFR 312.62(b)]

Proper records in clinical trials are essential to demonstrate GCP and regulatory compliance.

The clinical investigator is required to keep detailed records of patient visits to demonstrate initial eligibility and continuous eligibility as well as all information regarding safety and efficacy.

We found two source documents signed and dated August 28, 2006, for Subject XX for Visit X. One of the source documents listed a non-qualifying mean X of X. The other source document listed a qualifying mean XX of X. The case report forms (CRFs) showed that the subject was initially randomized based on the non-qualifying XX of X.

This example typically represents the situation where several people collect data for a patient and thus enter different readings. Also, since the data was not examined thoroughly at the site—deficiency in data quality control—the errors were not properly addressed.

Subject XX withdrew from the study on March 30, 2006. However, an entry dated August 12, 2006 was made on the source record for the January 17, 2006 visit indicating that the subject did not smoke and/or consume alcohol.

Sometimes addressing errors or omissions in the data collected as required by the protocol, for example, after a long overdue monitoring visit occurs, may show the carelessness in recording important data for a study. In the sample above, we can observe that the investigator apparently forgot to include information on alcohol and tobacco consumption that may have been criteria for inclusion and, after a monitoring visit or internal quality check, decided to include that data as it was a key component on the decision to include a patient. Well, basically with this observation it is evident that the person(s) recording key data for the clinical trial was not aware of the importance of this information (lack of training?), monitoring was very limited, and data verification did not follow the principle of generating a proper audit trail.

No Case Report Forms were completed for subjects xx, yy, zz, and bb.

Clinical trial data is collected from the sources (patient files, charts, lab results, etc.) into case reports forms (CRFs). If a paper CRF is generated, a copy must remain at the site. That copy has to be retained for an established period and its disposition documented.

Protocol [redacted] required that each subject be instructed to take 4 capsules of study medication once a day, at the same time of day during the treatment period and that the dose was to be administered with 240 mL of water. The investigation found no documentation that such instructions were given and no record confirming that these requirements were met. ... Your May 31, 2007 response states the protocol did not provide instructions of how to ensure that 240 mL of water was consumed, or how to document this fact. This response is unacceptable. It is the responsibility of the clinical investigator to ensure that protocol specified procedures are followed and documented.

Although the investigator pointed out that the sponsor might not have provided specific instructions on the matter, here is a compliance issue that always affects the outcome of any treatment (investigational or not) where patients are dispensed study medication and instructions are provided verbally. Generally, for in patients, study nurses should keep this information together with the patient chart. For outpatients, IRB approved written instructions should be provided and drug accountability should be the tool for compliance. Of course, there would not be any evidence of the 240 mL of water taken for the outpatient but his/her word. Here, the investigator was puzzled as to the level of evidence the inspector required and the study sponsor did not address.

> For the [redacted] protocol, the concomitant medications required to be entered on the Concomitant Medication eCRF were not entered, and some source records were inconsistent with eCRF entries. Specifically, source records document that Subject [redacted] received Benicar, acetaminophen with codeine, rosiglitazone maleate with glimepiride (4 mg/2 mg), Premarin 1 g, oxybutynin 5 mg, and Toprol XL, whereas the Case Report Form documents only Benicar, Toprol XL, metformin, and oxybutynin 5 mg. Furthermore, the Date Started column is not completed, and initials of the reviewing physician are not recorded.

In collecting protocol-specified data, concomitant medication is very important since it may uncover a serious underlying condition or an exclusion. In entering concomitant medication, mainly medication the patient is actually taking but not have been prescribed, the investigator makes sure that there is no contraindicated medication in the list, and that the patient is not being treated outside the protocol for an other serious ailment. This data has to be collected precisely in each and every case.

> There were two subjects screened for #(XX) with the initials (XX) and both were screen fails. The records for these two subjects were mixed in the different folders and because of the way that the records are identified, it is difficult to discern which documents belong to which subject.

It is extremely important that the investigative site understand that study records must not only be kept, but they have to be legible and in order. Accessibility to those records is critical if important safety data must be verified or other serious issue arises. Observations regarding how the records are maintained can point at more serious issues such as the veracity of the same. Therefore, before the study starts, the investigator site should implement a recordkeeping system that will comply with all requirements and also be easily accessible and retrievable.

The worst case scenario is when records are rewritten and "adjusted" to show compliance as follows:

> A new PK (pharmacokinetic) sample preparation record was made for Subject [XX] and the original was discarded with no adequate explanation. Information on the original record had been questioned by the sponsor's monitor, and based on a November 2, 2006 monitoring letter, the newly created record contained information that was previously not present on the original record. Specifically, a letter from the sponsor monitor dated October 10, 2006 stated that the [XX] sample at Week 4 for Subject [XX] was marked not done in the eCRF, but the source PK log was completed stating the centrifugation time and processing details for the sample. Per the monitor's request, the sample processing information on the PK log was deleted during the visit, and this change was initialed and dated. However, following the next monitoring visit, the monitor pointed out in a November 2, 2006 letter that the PK log for Subject [XX] was not the same log she saw at the previous monitoring visit. The monitor wrote that the changes she witnessed at the previous visit were missing from the newly created log, and the [XX] sample was labeled as "not done" on the new log. The newly created log also contained all the PK processing information which was noted as missing at the previous monitoring visit. This

PK processing information was not found in the subject records, although it is crucial source documentation. In your October 8, 2007 response letter, you acknowledged that the original log was created, and stated that the original was discarded as it was "illegible" due to a coffee spill. You also stated that you have addressed this issue with your staff. However, you did not provide an adequate explanation for the new information contained on the newly created log that had not been present on the original record.

This observation is very serious from many perspectives. First, the investigator using electronic CRFs (eCRFs) should be exercising extreme care when entering data and should ascertain that only internally verified data is entered. Therefore, a procedure should exist either in the protocol or at the site. The other issue is that the eCRF notes that PK sample at Week 4 was not done. If data exists on the time and processing details on that sample at Week 4, the reasonable step should have been to request from the lab that analyzed the sample confirmation of the existence of such. If it is confirmed, it means that the information entered in the eCRF is wrong and electronic data resolution should have been done for the eCRF field. If the lab analyzing the sample confirms that the sample does not exist, then with that information a correction in the log should be created and documented. The investigator should have been informed as to how to properly correct erroneous data in records, and if for any reason a record has to be made legible, the original should be kept for reference. Moreover, the investigator should also have confirmatory documents to support any correction to his/her records before it is made.

The investigator should record data as it is generated. The study coordinator or assisting qualified personnel should also be informed that any record alteration should be signed and dated. *A record should never be backdated (or forward dated)*, and all provisions should be made to utilize properly qualified personnel to enter and acknowledge data. The following is a clear example of having investigator site juggle compliance:

For Subject [XX] visit on August 31, 2006, source and progress notes appear to have been written and signed by a study coordinator, but the study coordinator was not at the office that day. In your October 8, 2007 response letter, you acknowledged that the study coordinator was hospitalized at the time, and you and another staff member performed the subject's visit. Additionally, you acknowledged that the study coordinator back-dated the notes to the day of the visit rather than the day the notes were written. You note that you addressed this issue with your staff, and we acknowledge that you wrote a Note to File to clarify that the progress note was actually written on September 5, 2006.

To maintain adequate and reliable records of a clinical investigation is part of the record requirement. The other part is retention for the required period of time as per GCP and the FDA. The most prominent observation in this matter is as follows:

You failed to retain records required to be maintained by the clinical investigator under 21 CFR part 312 for a period of 2 years following the date a marketing application is approved for the drug for the indication for which it is being investigated; or, if no application is to be filed or if the application is not approved for such indication, until 2 years after the investigation is discontinued and FDA is notified [21 CFR 312.62(c)]. . . .

Your failure to retain records of this clinical study makes it impossible for FDA to verify the integrity of the data and to verify that there was adequate protection of the rights, welfare, and safety of the subjects who participated in the study.

Findings Relating to the Investigational Product in Clinical Trials

(1) You failed to maintain investigational drug disposition records with respect to use by subjects. [21 CFR 312.62(a)]

This observation, despite being a records issue, pertains to the accountability of the investigational product. The investigator must keep detailed accountability records of the investigational product entrusted to him/her by the sponsor. Every dose must be properly accounted for and disposed of according to protocol. It is a serious finding that the accountability of the investigational product is not properly maintained.

In Protocol, the drug accountability logs for Subjects x, y, z could not be found. We acknowledge that in your Undated Letter you stated that you maintained drug accountability logs in the past only if the sponsor had provided one.

Proper accountability is part of the requirements of 21 CFR 312. Every well-trained investigator should be aware that accountability records logs, if not provided by the sponsor, have to be kept internally at the site.

Regarding study xx, a report dated 7/20/04 to the Data Safety Monitoring Board (DSMB) and IRB indicated that the [XX] made an error by including placebo capsules in a bottle that should have contained only the investigational drug. The report indicated that this involved one subject for a period of one week, during which the subject received between 50 and 90% of the correct investigational drug. A memorandum dated 4/20/04 describes a dispensing error in medication on 2/17/04 when capsules were dispensed for subjects [XX].

This finding indicates that the site unnecessarily delayed reporting of a dispensing error, which could significantly affect the safety of patients.

Protocol [redacted] Section 4.5.8, states "Drug administration will be documented (date, time, dose and signature of dispensing person). Drug account of the unused study medication will be performed." The investigation found that the Drug Dispensing log entries for 14 subjects who completed the study as of March 2007 contained incomplete information and did not adequately account for subject compliance. For example:

(a) For Subject [redacted] the Drug Dispensing log documents that the amount of drug used was "unknown" with no explanation provided for the lack of drug accountability.

It is investigator's responsibility to ensure that the study medication is taken only by eligible patients and that proper accountability as to how many doses were taken is performed. We must account for every dose received, dispensed, and returned. The person who conducts the accountability audit has to be held responsible for the task, and sign and date each record. Only properly qualified personnel should be engaged in drug dispensing and accountability.

(b) For Subject [redacted] the Drug Dispensing log documents the number of tablets and injections administered as unknown and that the patient never returned study medication.

The investigator must ensure that a patient, to whom study medication was effectively dispensed, returns the unused medication regardless of whether that patient completed the study or withdrew. The investigator must provide evidence of all efforts to recover unused medication from dropped out or withdrawn patients.

(c) For Subject [redacted] the Drug Dispensing log documents that 21 tablets and 16 injections were administered to the subject and that the subject returned 19 tablets, with no explanation provided in the "discrepancy" column.

This subject failed to take study medication. Therefore, the investigator must ensure that when a patient returns medication, if discrepancies appear, they must be clarified as to the reason of the discrepancy.

These drug accountability discrepancies are an example of clinical trial site inaccuracies in complex clinical trials where extensive monitoring should have captured them easily.

The other factor of why it is so important to provide for proper drug accountability is to detect lack of compliance. It is reasonable to assume that if we have evidence that the patient did not take medication, that his/her symptoms will continue and we can expect lack of efficacy. Accountability records will also allow a sponsor to determine the exclusion/inclusion of a patient in the final efficacy analysis. It is not possible to assure compliance if drug accountability records are not accurate.

Both the original protocol and Protocol Amendment #1 specified that [XX] vials were to be refrigerated at [XX] and should remain refrigerated until just prior to use. Our inspection found that there were no records found prior to January 2007 to confirm that the study medication was stored appropriately per the protocol requirements.

The investigator is required to store the investigational product according to protocol requirements until it is dispensed to patients. Proper temperature and humidity logs have to be maintained at all times to demonstrate that the product was stored under conditions determined to ensure stability. Failure to do so may compromise the reliability of the data, since there is no evidence that the product was in the condition established by the sponsor. Additionally, the investigator should have documentation to evidence that the temperature and humidity conditions established in the protocol for the investigational product received were maintained during transport.

Findings Relating to the Reporting of Adverse Events

(2) You failed to promptly report to the IRB all unanticipated problems involving risk to human subjects or others. (21 CFR 312.66)

The investigator also has responsibilities toward the institutional review board that approved the study at the site such as reporting serious adverse events.

In Protocol XX, your site was informed on December 12, 2006 that Subject X had been admitted to the hospital for a bilateral pulmonary embolism on [date], and had remained in the intensive care unit for one week. You failed to notify the IRB per IRB requirements within three business days of becoming aware of this serious adverse event, and you reported this event to the IRB on February 12, 2007 as a protocol deviation rather than an adverse event.

and

In your Undated Letter, you noted in response that Ms. [XX] was the primary study coordinator for this protocol. This response is inadequate, because your site became aware of this event after Ms. [XX] employment termination from your site. In addition, [XY], rather than Ms. [XX], made this notation after speaking to the subject on December 12, 2006.

This finding points out different issues regarding the investigator's understanding of his/her obligations and protocol adherence that resulted in the misreporting of a serious adverse event (SAE). The investigator did not have a proper procedure implemented for immediating reporting to him/her any serious adverse event suffered by a patient. In addition, since the study staff failed to notify the investigator of the event immediately, the SAE report to the IRB was delayed, a compliance issue. This particular finding points at the fact that the site personnel were not adequately trained to perform all clinical trial duties in a compliant manner.

Underreporting of adverse events is a serious finding since it can jeopardize the credibility of the data for the entire study, as follows:

The [redacted] protocol required that all adverse events be fully recorded on the subject's Case Report Form. The investigation found clinic records that documented loss of memory, and isolated nonobstructive thrombus in the common femoral vein on the right side for Subject [redacted] on November 28, 2006; left foot drop for Subject [redacted] on December 7, 2006; and urinary incontinence for Subject [redacted] on January 12 and 14, 2007. These adverse events were not documented onto the subjects' Case Report Form . . . . Your May 24, 2007 response states these adverse events were documented in the subject's medical history and physical examination report. This response is insufficient, as these adverse events were required to be documented on the subjects' Case Report Form.

Regardless of the seriousness or relationship to the study treatment, all adverse events have to be reported on the case report forms (CRFs) that are the required formats for clinical trial data. The data from those CRFs will ultimately be entered into the database and analyzed. Therefore, all adverse events must be included. If space is not provided on the CRFs, a proper written letter should be sent to the sponsor regarding the issue. If the sponsor is the same as the investigator, he/she should reevaluate the issue and document it immediately.

The [XX] protocol excluded female subjects who "are not using adequate birth control method." The protocol lists birth control pills or barrier method as the only acceptable means for birth control. The investigation found that Subject [XX] who was 18 years of age at the time, was "encouraged" to practice abstinence for at least three months after having the surgical procedure (December 2006). Furthermore, the investigation found that this subject had been previously scheduled to undergo surgery (May 15, 2006), but was found to have become pregnant and underwent abortion. . . . Your response letter dated May 18, 2007 states that you received sponsor approval for allowing this subject to use abstinence as a form of birth control. This response is unacceptable. An email dated April 5, 2007 from [XX] Medical Research Associate [XX] instructed the staff to discuss only the protocol specified birth control options with this subject.

In dissecting this observation, there are several issues that have to be stressed. In all clinical trials where female patients with childbearing potential are included, proven methods of contraception are recommended to avoid unnecessary risk of exposing a fetus to an investigational product. Methods such as the birth control pill or the barrier method alone, in my opinion, although methods of contraception, may also fail. Specifically, the birth control pill, if taken together with an investigational product, may fail to provide adequate contraception control due to possible drug interactions. Also, the barrier method utilized alone, if not properly used, does not provide adequate protection. Proven methods are IUDs, menopause, and hysterectomy, or if a barrier method is selected it should be used in conjunction with another contraceptive method such as foam, and still the failure rates are high.

In this particular case, where a young female patient had become unwittingly pregnant previously, more precautions should have been taken, and the patient should have been particularly advised of the protocol requirements that advise should have been documented. Nonetheless, the birth control pill should have been the chosen alternative in this case, if there is evidence that the study treatment will not make it less effective, since the barrier method alone is not as reliable. Abstinence may have been an option discussed with the patient; however, there is no documentation to suggest that. The investigator may have discussed this particular issue with the sponsor but failed to document it properly, and therefore the statement "you received sponsor approval for allowing this subject to use abstinence as a form of birth control" is not acceptable since there is no supporting documentation.

Also, let us examine the following portion of the letter: An email dated April 5, 2007 from [redacted] Medical Research Associate [redacted] instructed the staff to discuss only the protocol specified birth control options with this subject.

This patient underwent surgery on December 2006, almost 5 months before the medical research associate documented instructions for the particular patient. So this email only documents that the sponsor adhered to the protocol requirement *after* the fact and did not examine the investigator's "deviations."

> The original protocol and Protocol Amendment #1 specified that within one working day after a Serious Adverse Event, the investigator was to fill out and submit the SAE notification form. The information on the form was to include an evaluation of the relationship to the study drugs, and the form was also to be signed and dated. Per the written consultation report by Dr. [XX] dated July 27, 2006, your sub-investigator was aware that Subject [ZZ] had been admitted to the hospital with chest pains. During the hospital stay, a left heart catheterization, bilateral selective coronary angiogram and angioplasty were subsequently performed on the subject. You did not submit the initial report of the SAE to the sponsor (signed and dated by you) until December 5, 2006.

This is a clear example of delays in reporting SAEs according to protocol requirements. The requirement is that the investigator report SAEs as soon as he/she becomes aware of them. That means for this case on July 28, 2006. However, it took almost 5 months to have it formally reported. A significant delay in SAE reporting can jeopardize the safety of all patients in a clinical trial since that data is not available for evaluation by the data safety monitoring board appointed for that purpose and thus there will be unnecessary exposure of patients to an investigational product with such a profile.

Findings Relating to the Institutional Review Board's Approvals and Reporting

(1) You failed to assure that an Institutional Review Board (IRB) complying with applicable regulatory requirements was responsible for the continuing review and approval of a clinical study. (21 CFR 312.66)

It is the investigator's responsibility to ensure the continuing review and approval of clinical trials. It is very well known that institutional review boards may not issue a renewal automatically unless the investigator site submits an interim safety report together with the application for renewal, and the IRB meets to discuss the continuance of the study.

If for any reason the IRB did not issue a continuance of approval or reapproval, the site must suspend the study (this bears serious consequences). Therefore, no new patients can be enrolled since the IRB could not conclude that the study can continue safely.

You continued to perform research activities during timeframes when the IRB's study approval was expired. Examples include, but are not limited to, the following:

a. Study [XX] lapsed in IRB approval from 3/19/93 until 4/29/93. During this timeframe subject [XX] was enrolled (4/15/93). The study also lapsed in IRB approval from 7/14/95 until 9/28/95. During this timeframe subject [XX] was enrolled (7/18/95).

b. Study [XX] lapsed in IRB approval from 6/30/05 until 9/08/05, and from 9/7/06 until 10/05/06. Subjects were receiving study medications or seen for evaluations during these time periods.

The previous example points out that requesting a continuation of approval or reapproval does not guarantee that the IRB will approve and that the study can be continued.

The investigator site should be aware that it must request reapproval from the IRB well in advance according to the IRB performance history so that continuance of the study is ensured.

(2) You continued to conduct clinical investigation related activities despite the fact that IRB approval had been withdrawn. [21 CFR 312.66 and 56.103(a)]

Here is an example:

Despite your awareness of the withdrawal of IRB approval per the notice you received on May 11, 2005, you continued to obtain informed consent or parental consent from 27 of the 33 subjects previously entered into the study after May 12, 2005. Although [redacted] Human Research Board denied the request for you to conduct six-month and twelve-month follow up visits on May 22, 2005, six-month study visits were completed for six study subjects during the period that the clinical investigation was suspended by the IRB.

It is very important to understand that if an IRB approval is suspended for any reason, no new patients can be entered into a study, no new consents can be signed, no medication can be dispensed, all medication has to be collected, and enrolled patients must be terminated by assigning a proper follow-up therapy.

Moreover, the following was noted:

> In your written response, you stated that you did not know you were not permitted to conduct follow up visits after approval had been withdrawn.

The investigator is responsible for the health and well-being of patients during the study and the assigned follow-up period. Once the study is suspended by either party, the investigator continues to have responsibility for the health and welfare of the patients: that is for standard medical treatment not for the purpose of clinical trial. Also, if during the established follow-up period a patient of a suspended trial reports adverse events or serious adverse events, those still have to be reported to the sponsor and the IRB and treated accordingly.

To make things more complicated, the following was noted:

> Our investigation found that after having the clinical investigation reinstated by the IRB in September of 2005, you failed to notify the IRB that you were discontinuing the study in February 2006 and failed to submit a final study report. We find your explanation that you thought this was the sponsor's responsibility to be unacceptable.

After all the issues the investigator had in having the clinical trial suspension withdrawn, he/she decided to withdraw from the study. It is important to note that the investigator may also terminate his/her participation in a study with a properly documented reason. At that point, the investigator has the obligation to communicate that reason to the IRB that approved the study.

Note that the investigator is the only party that communicates with the IRB; therefore, sending a final report to the board at the conclusion of the study is an inherent responsibility.

(3) You failed to promptly report to the IRB all changes to the research activity and failed to promptly report all unanticipated problems involving risk to human subjects. (21 CFR 312.66)

Let us examine the following:

> You failed to promptly notify the IRB that Study 2 was placed on clinical hold. In your absence, FDA notified subinvestigation [XX] on 9/25/03 that the study was placed on clinical hold, and FDA sent you a letter dated 10/17/03 listing the clinical hold issues. You did not inform the IRB about the clinical hold until 1/2/04, when you submitted a protocol amendment and revised consent form.

This is a serious issue regarding personal supervision by the investigator during a study and delegation of responsibilities. Although a subinvestigator was assigned to a study during the principal investigator's absence, that delegate was not aware of regulatory and reporting requirements to the IRB, and therefore proper halt of a study was not implemented, subsequently endangering the enrolled patients.

> You failed to promptly report the unexpected adverse events experienced by the study subjects to the IRB as shown in the following examples....The IRB approval letter dated 9/1/99 for Study 1 required you to report any unexpected event experienced by the subjects within 24 hours followed by a written report within 10 working days of the event. You did not report the unexpected adverse event of increase in transaminases experienced by subject [XX] on 4/4/00 until 5/19/00, nearly six weeks after the adverse

event occurred. We note that you revised the consent form to include the additional risk of increased liver enzymes based on this adverse event.

IRBs may have their own reporting requirements for SAEs that are not always aligned with regulatory timelines. Also, IRBs may have their own forms and therefore the investigator should use them as appropriate. In collecting this information, IRBs also fulfill their own responsibilities.

Findings Relating to the Investigator Acting in a Dual Role of Sponsor–Investigator Investigators who also assume the sponsor's responsibilities are at high risk of noncompliance if they are not properly aware of the regulatory requirements. Findings range from not obtaining proper FDA approvals to lacking monitoring and quality assurance. Investigators who perform their own studies within medical institutions or academia may not have access to regulatory support and quality assurance as commercial sponsors do. Findings in these cases are more conspicuous.

(a) You allowed subjects to participate in an investigation without FDA approval. [21 CFR 812.110(a)]

Let us examine the following:

A physician that conducts an investigation, which is defined as a clinical investigation or research involving one or more subjects to determine the safety or effectiveness of a device, 21 CFR 812.3(h), with a device for an indication that has not been FDA-approved or cleared shall not allow subjects to participate in the investigation [21 CFR 812.110(a)].... This clinical investigation of the safety and effectiveness of a new indication for the [XX] requires an FDA-approved IDE. You allowed subjects to participate in the investigation without FDA approval.

This is a clear example of the principle that any clinical investigation that takes the form of a clinical trial to examine the safety and efficacy of a product (device, drug, biologic, etc.) and has a protocol and collects data in an organized manner for further analysis must be approved by the FDA prior to being initiated (FDA-regulated studies). The rationale behind this is that the function of the FDA is to determine that the rights, safety and well-being of human subjects who take part in the clinical investigation are protected. This applies to any study regardless of the intent to submit for a market application in the future.

(b) Failure to ensure proper monitoring of the investigation, obtain IRB review and approval, submit an IDE application to FDA, receive FDA approval of the IDE before beginning the investigation, and control devices under investigation. [21 CFR 812.100, 21 CFR 812.110(a), 21 CFR 812.40 and 21 CFR 812.42]

Essentially, once the clinical investigator assumes the responsibility of the sponsor, he/she should know and understand the regulatory implications of running clinical trials. Once the investigator fails to submit for regulatory approval, he/she fails to adhere to all responsibilities of an investigator and sponsor.

The sponsor–investigator duality role is very complicated and investigators should be made aware of this by their institutions. In the case of medical devices, oversights are more evident since there is a provision that, for Class II nonsignificant risk devices, FDA approval is not required (IDE), but IRB submission and approval is required. However, the misstep is when an investigator decides to classify the device by him/herself without taking into consideration all provisions for risk classification, or leaving it to the IRB personnel who may not have proper training in regulatory requirements for device risk classification. The device classification is done taking into account several factors: the safety of the use of a device in nonapproved indications where the risk to the patient is very high (e.g., in any implantable device where surgery is necessary). Therefore, regardless of the fact that an IDE or PMA seems unnecessary, the FDA should be contacted to determine the proper classification. Subsequently, the sponsor–investigator, with proper FDA risk classification documentation, can proceed with the clinical investigation.

4.2   AN ANALYSIS OF WARNING LETTERS ISSUED TO CLINICAL TRIAL SPONSORS AND THE IMPACT ON PRODUCT DEVELOPMENT

When clinical research sponsors are mentioned, we assume that commercial sponsors or the pharmaceutical industry is involved. However, sponsors may be the investigators or third parties that assumed the responsibility to develop an investigational product. In this section we deal with the sponsor's responsibilities in the matter.

Pharmaceutical sponsors, generally, have stronger regulatory and quality assurance resources to remain compliant in clinical trials and serious findings are not as common. However, there are still sponsor noncompliance issues, mainly when the sponsor is also the investigator or a medical device company.

4.2.1   Most Common Sponsors of Clinical Investigations Findings

Findings Relating to the Sponsor's Responsibilities to Ensure Proper Monitoring of a Clinical Trial

(a) You failed to monitor the progress of all clinical investigations being conducted under your IND. [21 CFR 312.56(a)]

Let us examine the following:

The FDA inspection disclosed that you did not maintain any documentation to indicate that the above studies conducted under an IND were adequately monitored. In your August 13, 2008 response letter to the Form FDA 483, you stated that you were personally involved in the care and treatment of every subject and treatment of every subject who participated in the [XX] studies at the University, and monitored their progress. You stated that during the last several years, a DSMB monitored the data collected during the studies to assure patient safety. You stated that it is true that you relied on individuals at the University [XX] to help assure that the research was properly conducted in [city], and on a colleague at an academic institution in [XX] to do the same at his site. However, you acknowledged that you failed to document monitoring activities adequately.

This is a case where the investigator also assumes the responsibility of the sponsor. He/she must ensure that there is adequate monitoring of the study and must document it properly with, for example, monitoring reports. Regardless of whether the sponsor is a commercial enterprise or not, the monitoring requirement is not overridden. Universities or other academic institutions may not be able to provide regulatory and monitoring support for a clinical site; therefore, reliance on the institution may not be appropriate.

> This inspection revealed an absence of monitoring of clinical activities at the [XX] Cancer Center. In your letter to the FDA (Enclosure B), you stated that patients seen at [XX] Cancer were carefully monitored. However, during the inspection, there were multiple examples of the lack of monitoring activities resulting in a direct impact on the conduct of the clinical trials and the safety of human subjects.

This is a case where the sponsor–investigator interprets "adequate monitoring" as medical monitoring of the patient's status. The lack of understanding of the regulatory requirement of the sponsor's responsibility to monitor clinical trial activities in addition to monitoring the patient status yields all types of monitoring observations (e.g., lack of monitoring personnel, lack of monitoring reports, lack of control of the quality of data entered on the CRFs).

(b) Failure to secure investigator compliance with the investigational plan and applicable FDA regulations. [21 CFR 312.56(b)]

Let us examine the following:

> Review of [XX] monitoring records, [XX] Quality Assurance (QA) audit records, and email communications between [CRO] and [sponsor] disclosed that [sponsor] knew of pervasive problems at the clinical investigator site of Dr. [bb], a solo practitioner in rural Alabama who had never previously conducted an FDA-regulated study, but randomized 407 subjects into Study 3014 over a 3 month time period (i.e., November 2001–January 2002.). . . . We note that [sponsor] failed to promptly secure compliance from Dr. [bb] and did not adequately investigate allegations of fraud at this site.

This is a serious observation directed at the sponsor of a clinical trial. Strong evidence suggests that compliance has been compromised and patient safety jeopardized. The sponsor failed to properly address the issue in a satisfactory manner, such as scrutinizing the data provided by the investigator immediately, and suspended the site until a formal investigation could be conducted. Moreover, the sponsor failed to notify the FDA of the serious observations that may further compromise the validity of the data for the market application.

> Our review has disclosed that despite periodic clinical monitoring visits made by, or on behalf of, your firm, serious protocol violations were repeatedly made by several of the participating clinical investigators. For example, between October 14, 1996, and March 27, 1998, [sponsor] made a total of 16 monitoring visits. . . . Review of sponsor/monitor records, as well as those collected during FDA's April 1998 data audit of this clinical investigator, disclosed that protocol violations continued throughout this period.

This observation points to serious oversights. The sponsor had monitored the study and issued reports. However, the quality of monitoring and assurance is questioned in this finding, where the sponsor did not prove that it took any action on protocol violations but only reported them.

For example, the inspection revealed the following:

> It also was noted that [XX] failed to observe the protocol with regard to the administration of a study-related medication. . . . The investigational plan required. . . .be initiated during the 24-hour period preceding stenting. However, none of the 31 subjects in the SCORES trial at this site received [XX] prior to the stenting procedure. . . . should have adhered to the protocol. The sponsor was aware of this clinical investigator's objection to the protocol's regimen and the resulting protocol deviations, yet it did not secure Dr. [bb's] compliance.

This is a particular example of failing to ensure compliance by the investigator site. The sponsor has the obligation to ensure compliance and therefore has to demonstrate that all investigative sites follow the protocol. If violations or deviations are observed during monitoring visits, the sponsor should address those with the investigator and make sure that they are not repeated by documenting all actions. Also, the sponsor must ensure that the IRBs are notified. Failure to implement corrective actions may jeopardize the data from the site and the entire study. If an investigator does not agree with protocol procedures, he/she must address those in writing, and if a solution is not achieved, the sponsor should terminate that site and notify the FDA.

(c) Failure to possess written monitoring procedures and failure to ensure proper monitoring of the investigation. [21 CFR 812.25(e) and 21 CFR 812.40]

Let us examine the following:

> You failed to provide written monitoring procedures for monitoring the study. The [XX] does not include monitoring procedures (i.e., monitoring schedule, adherence to protocol, verification of source documents to case report forms) for monitoring the study. In addition, you were not able to provide monitoring correspondence or reports, therefore you failed to ensure proper monitoring of the investigation.

Monitoring is a sponsor's responsibility according to GCP and regulatory requirements. All sponsors of clinical trials regardless of the investigational product must assure that the studies are properly monitored to ensure patient safety and data validity. Failure to monitor may render the data obtained of uncertain quality.

> The frequency of monitoring visits at study sites deviated considerably from the monitoring plan that your firm established. In addition, [sponsor's] own "Clinical Research Standard Operating Procedures" for this study state that visits will be performed at intervals determined necessary to ensure compliance with the investigational plan. This was not done.

This is a case where, from the procedural point of view, all documentation was available to ensure compliance but, from the implementation point of view, the sponsor failed to follow their own procedures and therefore was found to be noncomplaint. Basically, the sponsor shoots his own foot.

(d) [Sponsor] failed to adequately monitor the clinical study as required by its monitoring guidelines. [as adopted August 9, 1994]

Let's us examine the following:

Monitoring guidelines require a review of the CRFs and 100 percent cross check of source documents for completeness and accuracy. However, FDA inspection of Dr. [XX] revealed that he did not maintain adequate and accurate source documents and other data pertinent to the administration of the investigational drug to study subjects or the control group.

This observation points out that it is not enough for the sponsor to have SOPs for monitoring; evidence must show that the monitoring of the study was compliant to both SOPs and regulatory requirements. This observation was prompted by an inspection of a sponsor once an investigator site inspection showed serious findings. The site did not have source documents, and used the CRFs as the source. Therefore, how did the monitor monitor?

Findings Relating to the Sponsor's Responsibilities for the Investigational Product

(a) **You failed to maintain adequate records showing the shipment of the investigational drug.** [21 CFR 312.57(a)]

Let us examine the following:

Regarding study [XX], during the inspection you did not have any documentation showing the shipment of investigational drugs to the clinical investigator at the [XX] site.

The sponsor is responsible for maintaining adequate documentation on the use and disposition of the investigational product, including detailed shipping records on who received study medication and the exact amount of doses shipped along with conditions of the shipment (temperature, humidity, etc., if applicable).

(b) **You failed to have an IND in effect prior to shipping the investigational new drug to investigators.** [21 CFR 312.20(b) and 312.40(c)]

Let us examine the following:

Your IND went into effect on June 7, 1996, but you shipped in ... 1994 to Dr. .... to conduct a 12 subject study.

Investigational product can only be shipped to an investigator site if the study has a valid IND and is approved by the IRB of the site once the sponsor initiated the study. Otherwise, the sponsor may run into serious noncompliance issues of shipping investigational products to nonqualified investigators (without IRB approval), or failing to verify that the site complies with all the requirements to start a study (though an initiation report).

Findings Relating to the Sponsor's Records of a Clinical Investigation

(a) **You failed to retain records for the requisite time period.** [21 CFR 312.57(c)]

Let us examine the following:

21 CFR 312.62(c) requires that a sponsor retain the records and reports required by 21 CFR Part 312 for 2 years after a marketing application is approved for the drug; or, if an application is not approved for the drug, until 2 years after shipment and delivery of the drug for investigational use is discontinued and FDA has been so notified.

It is important that record retention follows the minimum required period to allow inspectors to confirm adherence to regulatory requirements, to assure that patients' safety has not been compromised and the study demonstrates data quality and integrity.

Findings Relating to the Sponsor Obtaining an IND to Conduct a Study

(c) Failure to submit an Investigational New Drug Application (IND) to the FDA and failure to withhold administration of an investigational new drug until an IND is in effect. (21 CFR 312.20 and 312.50)

The sponsor must ensure that a proper IND application was filed and that the investigators are provided with the IND number.

Your firm administered investigational products, including [XX] and [XY] to human subjects without filing an IND. You co-author on articles published in medical journals with data from these studies, which were supported by government grants. . . . Seventy-two subjects were given radiolabel doses of [XX] without an IND in effect.

In this case where the investigator is also the sponsor of a clinical trial, it is imperative that the sponsor–investigator same be aware of regulatory requirements for clinical studies. This type of observation is seldom found in commercially sponsored studies, where proper regulatory support exists.

Findings Relating to the Sponsor's Responsibilities to Secure Agreements Within Parties

(b) You failed to obtain an investigator statement, Form FDA 1572, before permitting an investigator to participate in an investigation. [21 CFR 312.53(c)(1)]

Let us examine the following:

You allowed a clinical investigator to participate in the investigation prior to obtaining a signed investigator statement containing:

a. The name and address of the investigator;
b. The name and code number, if any, of the study(ies) in the IND identifying the study(ies) to be conducted by the investigator;
c. The name and address of any medical school, hospital, or other research facility where the clinical investigation(s) will be conducted;
d. The name and address of any clinical laboratory facilities to be used in the study;
e. The name and address of the IRB that is responsible for review and approval of the study(ies);
f. A commitment by the investigator that he or she:

   i. Will conduct the study(ies) in accordance with the relevant, current study(ies) and will only make changes in a study after notifying the sponsor, except when necessary to protect the safety, the rights, or welfare of subjects;

   ii. Will comply with all requirements regarding the obligations of clinical investigators and all other pertinent requirements in this part;

   iii. Will personally conduct or supervise the described investigation(s);

   iv. Will inform any potential subjects that the drugs are being used for investigational purposes and will ensure that the requirements relating to obtaining informed consent (21 CFR part 50) and institutional review board review and approval (21 CFR part 56) are met;

   v. Will report to the sponsor adverse experiences that occur in the course of the investigation(s) in accordance with 312.64;

   vi. Has read and understands the information in the investigator's brochure, including the potential risks and side effects of the drug; and

   vii. Will ensure that all associates, colleagues, and employees assisting in the conduct of the study(ies) are informed about their obligations in meeting the above commitments.

The sponsor of an investigation has the obligation to obtain the signed and dated FDA Form 1572 and submit it to the FDA. That form is a "contract" between the investigator and the FDA where the investigator assumes the mentioned responsibilities and that the clinical trial is going to be conducted according to 21 CFR 312. The sponsor cannot initiate a study (conduct the site initiation visit) unless this form is completed and the information is satisfactory.

(c) Failure to obtain an adequate signed investigator agreement for each participating investigator. [21 CFR 812.43(c)(5)]

In the case of medical devices, although there is no requirement for FDA Form 1572, the sponsor must obtain a signed agreement with the investigator.

> Pursuant to 21 CFR 812.43(c), a sponsor is required to obtain from each participating investigator a signed agreement that shall include sufficient accurate financial disclosure information to allow the sponsor to submit a complete and accurate certification or disclosure statement to FDA. The agreement also must contain a commitment from the investigator to promptly update this information if any relevant changes occur during the course of the investigation and for 1 year following the completion of the study.... You failed to obtain a signed investigator agreement from [XX] and [XX] that includes financial disclosure information.

4.3 ANALYSIS OF WARNING LETTERS ISSUED TO INSTITUTIONAL REVIEW BOARDS AND THE IMPACT ON PRODUCT DEVELOPMENT

Institutional review boards have the responsibility to approve clinical trials that will be conducted at the study site. Their responsibilities were initially summarized in the Declaration of Helsinki.

IRBs have not been very thorough with their approach to compliance. The observations made by the FDA point at a general failure to recognize their responsibilities and the implications for patient safety and data integrity. The IRBs are stakeholders together with the investigator and the sponsor in clinical research and proper understanding of their responsibilities will produce a compliant approval process.

Remember that an IRB that is not compliant to FDA (21 CFR 56) and GCP requirements cannot issue a valid approval. For an investigator, this is equivalent to no approval at all.

From inspected IRBs, serious violations were observed again and again. Commonly, unless part of commercial enterprises, IRBs are part of institutions and therefore seem to lack expert regulatory input to guide them in the compliance process. There is no certification or any qualifying process for IRBs or their members. However, the FDA implemented an IRB registration requirement, and all IRBs must comply with the initial registration requirement and, if necessary, make required revisions to their registrations by September 14, 2009. The purpose is to compile a comprehensive list of IRBs involved in reviewing clinical investigations regulated by the FDA.

4.3.1 Most Common Institutional Review Board Findings

Findings Relating to IRB Operational Procedures

(a) **Failure to prepare, maintain, and follow written procedures.** [21 CFR 56.108(a) and (b) and 56.115(a)(6)]

Let us examine the following:

Our inspectional review revealed that [XX] Eye Institute IRB does not have an official IRB written procedure. Examples of your failure to satisfy these requirements include but are not limited to the following: there is no documentation of any IRB handbook or bylaws in place; and there are no documents which define the authority, functions, operations, details, and other requirements of the board.

This finding is very disturbing, since IRBs have had responsibilities and requirements assigned by the regulation for more than two decades. Also, the initial guide of the Declaration of Helsinki should have prompted the IRB to formalize its activities. How should the IRB function and according to which standards and procedures should the activities be inspected?

(b) **The IRB failed to follow its written procedures for conducting the review of research, including periodic review.** [21 CFR 56.108(a)]

Let us examine the following:

Those policies required the IRB to assign a new tracking number to [XX] proposed new studies, and required full committee review. However, the IRB did not notice that the studies represented different studies using different investigational devices and sponsors. As a result, the IRB approved those studies incorrectly as continuations of a previously approved study under the same tracking number. Consequently, studies were conducted at your institution without proper review and approval.

The IRB is responsible for thorough review of the study protocol and other study-related material, from which it can assert if a new study is a continuation of a previously approved one.

(c) The written procedures do not adequately meet the regulatory requirements of 21CFR 56.108(b) and 21 CFR 56.115(a)(6).

Let us examine the following:

The IRB's written procedures entitled, "The [IRB] Community Hospital I.R.B. Manual," lack the following procedures: for determining which projects need verification from sources other than the investigator that no material changes have occurred since previous IRB review; for ensuring prompt reporting to the IRB, appropriate institutional officials and the FDA of instances of serious or continuing noncompliance of investigators with the regulations or the requirements of the IRB; for ensuring prompt reporting to the FDA of unanticipated problems including risks to human subjects; for determining "Significant Risk" (SR) versus "Non-significant Risk" (NSR) for medical device investigations.

or

The IRC functions under written procedures found in the Medical Staff Bylaws which were promulgated by the Medical Executive Committee. This document, adopted February 27, 1987, was last revised/updated in March 2003. These procedures do not meet the FDA requirements for written IRB procedures (i.e., providing sufficient detail regarding how review of research is conducted) in several areas. For example,

- There are insufficient details describing how the IRC conducts initial and continuing review of research studies. [See 21 CFR 56.108(a) and (b)]
- There are no procedures describing how the IRC determines the frequency for carrying out continuing review of studies, i.e., how the IRB identifies those studies that would require review more frequently than once a year. [See 21 CFR 56.108(a)]

This is essential for the investigator to know when and how to apply for continuing review.

- There is no procedure for handling expedited reviews/approvals, even though the IRC utilizes the expedited review process. (See 21 CFR 56.108(a) and 56.110)

The investigator should have access to all compliant IRB procedures if expedited review is necessary.

- There are no procedures for determining whether investigational device studies involve significant vs. nonsignificant risk devices. (See 21 CFR 56.108(a) and 812.66)

The IRB should decide on the risk classification of a device, since it may have further regulatory implications. Not having those procedures puts the investigator in jeopardy of having a nonvalid approval.

- The procedures lacked details concerning the minimum number of members needed to review and vote on approval of research studies, including the need for there to be at least one non-scientific member present.
- The Bylaws state that a quorum shall consist of $33\frac{1}{3}$ voting members, but in no event less than 3 voting members. If your IRC consists of 11 members, under FDA regulations, a quorum would be 6 members (50% + 1).

The IRB misinterpreted the quorum to such an extent that previously approved studies were put at risk.

- The IRC procedures do not address specifically how adverse events are handled. The approval notifications to investigators state only that any adverse events are to be reported to the IRC immediately, but lack additional details such as criteria for determining what constitutes an adverse event.

IRBs are required to obtain all safety information such as adverse events and serious adverse events in a clinical trial. That is part of the continuous review of the ongoing studies. Having procedures for reporting SAEs and/or an explanation of what constitutes an SAE forces the investigator to make reports using standard formats and according to the protocol established criteria.

It is important that, if an IRB reviews particular studies, it has the proper SOPs in place to be fully compliant with regulatory requirements, and that periodical review of those procedures is performed.

The [XX] laboratory submitted the new study entitled [XX] on 11/15/00. The IRB assigned the study tracking number of [XX] and approved the study on 2/05/01. Under the same tracking number, the clinical investigator later submitted an "amendment" to [XX] that was, in fact, a new protocol entitled [XX]. The IRB approved this "amendment" request via expedited review process on 3/11/02 without realizing that it was a new protocol that should have been assigned a new tracking number.

This finding indicates that the IRB was not able to follow its own procedure in identifing new protocols and reviewing them accordingly.

The written procedures do not contain a description of the qualifications for IRB membership or a statement as to the length of time the IRB records are to be maintained.

The above are requirements are part of 21 CFR 56.

The IRB has no procedures regarding studies that experience a lapse in IRB approval. For FDA-regulated studies, with the exception of activities necessary to ensure the welfare of the study subjects, no study-related activities are to occur during an approval lapse. The inspectional report notes that an adverse effect occurred in the [XX] study on [XX], during a lapse in IRB approval of this study, indicating that the study remained in progress despite the lapse in approval.

IRB approvals are valid for 1 year unless established otherwise for a shorter length due to the risk of the study. The investigator must resubmit for continuing approval before the original approval lapses in accordance to IRB SOPs. The IRB should have performance standards for the time it takes to review submitted documentation and those standards should be followed by the investigator. At the same time, the IRB should consider those studies that applied for continuing review in a commensurate manner to avoid lapse in approvals. Lapse means that the study must be suspended, no new patients enrolled, and the sponsor and IRB should be notified. Therefore, the investigator has to follow IRB procedures for those cases.

There is still a big question on the interpretation of 21 CFR 56 as to which procedures have to be written and implemented. For example,

There are no written procedures for the following activities:

- Review of research involving an exception from informed consent requirements for emergency research to ensure that the IRB has found and documented that specific criteria have been met and to ensure that additional protections of the rights and welfare of the subjects will be provided.
- How the IRC conducts its continuing review of research.
- How the IRC determines which projects require review more often than annually.
- How the IRC ensures that changes in approved research, during the periods for which IRC approval had already been given, are not initiated without IRC review and approval (except where necessary to eliminate apparent immediate hazards to subjects).
- How the IRC ensures prompt reporting to appropriate institutional officials and FDA of any instance of serious or continuing noncompliance.
- Review of research involving vulnerable populations such as pregnant women, prisoners, and minors.

Another example is the following:

The following written procedures do not comply with the requirements of 21 CFR Part 56:

- *Article V—Quorum* defines quorum as a majority of the committee members or four (4), whichever is less. 21 CFR 56.108(b) requires that a majority of members be present at convened meetings.
- *Article VIII — Expedited Review* states all studies submitted to the IRC shall be reviewed by the full committee, except for certain studies involving no more than minimal risk, for minor changes in research previously approved by the IRC, and for renewals of studies previously approved by the IRC. 21 CFR 56.110 does not allow for the expedited renewal of previously approved studies, but may be used for minor changes in previously approved research during the period of 1 year or less for which approval is authorized.
- *Article X— Records, Item C* defines a retention period of two years following the date of study completion. However, 21 CFR 56.115(b) requires that records be retained for at least 3 years after completion of the research.

- The IRC procedures cite the Federal Register dated Friday, November 11th, 1977, Part III as a reference for at least three of its procedures. This is an inappropriate reference because this is a Food and Drug Administration Final rule for the Investigational Device Exemption Requirements for Intraocular Lenses, 21 CFR Part 813, which has since been rescinded.

Findings Relating to IRB Initial and Continuing Review Process

Review of study documents indicates that the IRB failed to follow or failed to maintain written procedures for conducting initial and continuing review of research. For example: (a) The IRB failed to follow its written procedures for informed consent documents. Specifically, the IRB's procedures require that consents for medical research projects will contain specific required elements and additional elements. However, the consent form document approved for Study Protocol [XX] by the IRB on March 18, 2005, was missing the following elements that are required by your procedure: (i) a description of any reasonably foreseeable risks or discomforts to the subject; (ii) an explanation of whom to contact for answers to pertinent questions about the research and research subject's rights, and who to contact in the event of a research related injury to the subject.

It is very important that the IRB follows compliant procedures for the review process of clinical trial documents. The investigator should have those procedures available to assess compliance prior to submitting documents to the IRB for approval, since *the regulator puts the onus also on the investigator to have a compliant IRB review* the study documents.

(a) The IRB failed to conduct continuing review of research at intervals appropriate to the degree of risk. [21 CFR 56.109(f)]

Let us examine the following:

These new studies, which were approved as renewals and amendments incorrectly, should have been reviewed at least annually as required by the regulation.

IRBs are required to review studies at least once a year to determine that the study can proceed according to previous assessment, or a new risk assessment should be performed with the new safety information provided.

Review of study documents and related IRB minutes indicates that the IRB granted retroactive reapproval to two FDA-regulated studies, [XX] sponsored study of the use of [XX] and [XX]. The [XX] study was retroactively reapproved in both 2003 and 2004, after approximately two months of lapsed approval each time. The [XX] sponsored study was retroactively reapproved in 2003, also after approximately two months of lapsed approval.

Continuing review should be established in IRB compliant SOPs and the documentation should reflect the adherence to those procedures. Retroactive reapproval is not appropriate since this indicates that the investigator may not have applied on time or that the IRB took too long to review an application.

(b) Failure to prepare, maintain, and follow adequate written procedures designed to assure the protection of the rights and welfare of human subjects. [21 CFR 56.102(g), 56.108(a) and (b), 56.109(b), (c), and (d), and 56.115]

Continuing review of clinical trial activities at the institution where the IRB approved the studies is imperative to safeguard the health and welfare of subjects. Those reviews should be conducted at least once a year if the risk does not necessitate a more frequent review. The following finding explains deviations in the requirement.

According to *ARTICLE VI—MEETINGS* in the IRC's written procedures, contained in a document titled "INSTITUTIONAL REVIEW COMMITTEE BY-LAWS AND PHILOSOPHY," normal meetings will be held annually or as may be required at the call of the Chair, but not less frequently than annually. However, the IRC meeting minutes illustrate that this committee reviews research at convened meetings on a sometimes infrequent basis. As shown in the table below, convened meetings held from 2002 to 2008 did not always meet this requirement.

Findings Relating to IRB Recordkeeping and Retention

(a) The IRB failed to prepare and maintain adequate documentation of IRB activities. [21 CFR 56.115]

Let us examine the following:

The minutes of the IRB meetings do not document all actions taken by the IRB, and the vote on those actions, including the number of members voting for, against, and abstaining. The minutes from meetings on 3/21/02, 5/9/03, 7/18/03, 10/14/03, and 7/12/04 all failed to show the actions taken and the members voting for, against, and abstaining.

IRBs are required to maintain adequate minutes of meetings to document all discussions and actions taken. IRBs should always have a person assigned to take those minutes in a precise manner, since those are the only recorded evidence for board decisions and the reasons for those decisions.

For example,

Meeting minutes do not always record the basis for requiring changes in or disapproving research, and a summary discussion of controverted issues and their resolution. For example, the meeting minutes for the 07/18/03 meeting showed that eight new proposals, three annual renewals, and two amendments were approved without documenting the discussions and the basis for approval.

Also, a notable observation of limited recordkeeping is as follows:

For protocol [XX] "Phase I/II, Open-Label, Pharmacokinetic and Safety Study of a Novel [XX] the IRB sent a letter to the clinical investigator dated August 19, 2006 stating that the IRB reapproved the protocol. There is no mention of protocol [XX] in the minutes of the August 10, 2006 IRB meeting or in any other documentation. Therefore, due to the lack of adequate detail in the IRB meeting minutes and other documents, we are unable to confirm that the study was re-approved at a convened meeting as required by FDA regulations.

or

The IRC meeting minutes have not been prepared in sufficient detail to show the number of members voting for, against, and abstaining for the actions taken.

Any time an IRB meets to review clinical trials, detailed minutes of the meetings should be kept as to:

- Date and time the meeting is initiated
- Who attended the meeting, listing qualified members, and if quorum was reached
- Responsibilities of the voting members and other participants (consultants, etc.)
- Details on which clinical trial documents were reviewed (protocol versions and dates of issue, safety reports, consent forms) and new and resubmissions
- Review of expedited approvals, if applicable
- Comments of the members on the materials reviewed to document the discussions
- Record as to number of voting members who voted for, against, and abstained
- Decisions made on the documents reviewed
- Any other pertinent issues discussed
- Time meeting is adjourned

It is very important that the inspector has all elements to assess compliance to regulatory requirements and IRB SOPs.

(b) Failure to maintain copies of all research proposals reviewed. [21 CFR 56.115(a)(1)]

Let us examine the following:

Pursuant to 56.115(a)(1), an IRB is required to prepare and maintain adequate documentation of IRB activities including copies of all research proposals reviewed. The study protocol for the [XX] approved by the IRB on [XX] was not maintained in the IRB files. Apparently, the IRB maintained only the Request for Approval, the Protocol Summary, and correspondence for this study.

The IRBs are required to maintain records such as sponsors and investigators of all clinical trial related activities. At least one copy of each reviewed and approved document must be kept on file for the established period.

The worst case scenario applies to the following finding, where, besides having an IRB not complying with minimum recordkeeping procedures, the IRB also failed to understand applicable regulations as follows:

Your IRB's failure to have the required membership is evident by the fact that the IRB study files contain numerous approval letters to principal investigators of device studies in which the IRB requested, as part of its conditions for approval, the investigator's compliance with the Investigational New Drug (IND) regulations in 21 CFR Part 312 rather than the applicable Investigational Device Exemption (IDE) regulations in 21 CFR Part 812.

Other record findings include the following:

> The IRB failed to follow FDA regulations pertaining to review of research, which require that an IRB shall notify investigators and the institution in writing of its decision to approve or disapprove the proposed research activity, or of modifications required to secure IRB approval of the research activity [21 CFR 56.109(e)]. For protocol [XX] there is no documentation in the IRB's files that the investigator was notified of the October 3, 2005 approval of a Patient Information Sheet. In addition, on January 30, 2006, the clinical site submitted three documents to the IRB pertaining to Specimen Storage at Repositories funded by NICHD: (1) Information Sheet (Spanish and English); (2) Repository Consent Form for Parent (Spanish and English); and (3) Repository Consent Form For Youth (Spanish and English). There is no documentation that the investigator was notified of the approval of the consent forms.

Proper recordkeeping and documentation will ensure compliance. In this case there is no evidence that the documents were generated.

Findings Relating to IRB Composition and Membership

> The IRB failed to maintain records of the current members' earned degrees, representative capacity, indications of experience sufficient to describe each member's chief anticipated contribution to IRB deliberations, and any employment or other relationship between each member and the institution.

IRBs are required to maintain updated lists of their members, affiliations, and any conflict that they may have as investigators in clinical trials, such as vested interests in the sponsor companies. Those members have to be identified to further assess the objectivity of the review process.

> **(c) Failure to meet membership and/or quorum requirements.** [21 CFR 56.107(d), 56.108(c), and 812.60]

Let us examine the following:

> Examples of this failure include, but are not limited to, the following: The IRC has been reviewing and approving studies without a member unaffiliated with the institution since at least July 2000. The IRC meeting of May 29, 2002, did not meet quorum requirements in that only 4 of 11 members were present. Also, there was no non-scientist member present, as required by FDA regulations. Because the educational/professional background of [XX] was not documented, it is unclear if a "non-scientist" was present at the August 11, 2003, meeting.

In accordance with 21 CFR 56.107(a) and 56.107(d), each IRB is required to have at least five members with varying backgrounds, have members who are sufficiently qualified through experience, expertise, and diversity of interests, and have at least one member who is unaffiliated with the institution and not part of the immediate family of a person affiliated with the institution. Unless expedited review is being used, review of research must be conducted at meetings where a majority of IRB members are present, including at least one member whose primary concerns are in nonscientific areas [21 CFR 56.108(c)].

Records regarding each IRC member's representative capacity, indications of experience in sufficient detail to describe their anticipated contributions to IRC deliberations, and any employment or other relationship between each member and the institution are incomplete. IRC membership listings from July 1, 2000, to June 30, 2004, do not identify affiliation with the hospital for most members, and none of the members had CVs/resumes on file.

It is very important to have transparency in the process of review and approval of clinical trial protocols. The IRBs should have available a list of members and their affiliations as well as anticipated contributions to satisfy the investigator's need to determine that the IRB reviewing the study is duly constituted and compliant.

Findings Relating to IRB Review Process

(a) **The IRB failed to review proposed research at convened meetings at which a majority of the members of the IRB were present.** [21 CFR 56.108(c)]

It is very important that the IRB documents the listed members participating in a meeting and discusses and resolves issues *only* if a quorum is achieved.

For example,

According to the IRB's written procedures, the IRB consists of ten members, and the IRB Chair is not permitted to vote unless there is a tie. The section of IRB's policy entitled "IRB Chair's Duties, Authorities, and Responsibilities," under number 23, states that the IRB chair should "vote on IRB business only in case of a tie vote by the HSRC." The IRB failed to establish a majority of members at four meetings. On 3/21/03 and 5/19/03 there were five members in attendance, not including the IRB Chair. On 1/14/05 and 5/13/05 there were three and four members in attendance, respectively, not including the Chair. During the above days, the IRB voted to approve new studies, annual renewals, and amendments.

Obviously, the IRB failed to follow its own procedures.

The IRB allowed non-members to vote on research projects. The individuals listed in the table below voted during IRB meetings even though they were not listed on the IRB's membership roster for the corresponding time.

Only listed members with voting privileges are allowed to vote.

The IRB's procedures require that IRB meetings conducted by telephone are done in such a way that each participating member can actively and equally participate in the discussion, and that the minutes of such meetings clearly document that this condition has been met. The IRB failed to adhere to this procedure by conducting "voice votes" for approval of informed consent documents. These votes were conducted by means of an individual phone call to each IRB member by the IRB's Executive Assistant, with a request for their vote. For example: (i) The initial approval of the consent form for Study Protocol [XX] was approved by seven IRB members during a "special voice vote meeting" on March 18, 2005. There was no indication in the IRB records that any group discussion of the consent form occurred.

In the case that the IRB has a provision that meetings and discussions can be performed via telephone conference, evidence of discussion of the items reviewed is important to support compliance. The spirit of the regulation is to promote discussion on ethical aspects of a clinical trial.

(b) Failure to review proposed research at convened meetings at which a majority of the members of the IRB are present. [21 CFR 56.108(c)].

Mail ballot voting was used for all of the following approvals including the final approval to a study involving an exception from informed consent requirements for emergency research under 21 CFR 50.24. Except for expedited review of certain kinds of research involving no more than minimal risk, or minor changes in research; review of proposed research must be conducted at a convened meeting at which a majority of the membership of the IRB is present, including one member whose primary concerns are non-scientific. The use of a mail ballot to vote on issues before the IRB is not permitted because this method does not constitute a convened meeting.

This finding represents a critical deviation from the spirit of the requirement for discussion on the ethical considerations before issuing an approval or refusal. An IRB should be able to discuss all aspects of the protocol presented for review as well as all related documentation, including the patient information and consent form. From that discussion a real position of the members will be established and documented, to ensure the safety, rights, and well-being of subjects.

(c) Failure to fulfill requirements for expedited review. [21 CFR 56.110(b)(1)]

Let us examine the following:

An IRB may review certain research using an expedited review procedure if the research involves no more than minimal risk to subjects and/or there were minor changes in previously approved research during the period for which approval is authorized. The IRC Chair inappropriately used the expedited review process for continuing review of research.

For the case presented above, the IRB used the expedited review procedure that does not comply with 21CFR 56.110 (b)(1) since the approval was issued to grant continuance of a clinical trial.

(d) Failure to meet the requirements for review of research involving an exception from informed consent for emergency research. [21 CFR 56.109(c) and 50.24]

Let us examine the following:

For emergency research being conducted under 21 CFR 50.24, the IRB must also evaluate materials to determine whether the investigation satisfies the criteria in 21 CFR 50.24(a) and find and document whether it is appropriate to proceed under this section. Specifically, IRBs are expected to review plans for community consultation and public disclosure and must find and document that both of these will be provided prior to the start of the study. The [XX] Hospital IRC approved the [XX] study on 10/9/06 and failed to document that the study met the criteria set out in 21 CFR 50.24. Additionally, although the clinical investigator states that he conducted the community consultation and public disclosure activities, there is no documentation that the IRC evaluated these materials and determined that these additional protections would be provided prior to start of the study as required by 21 CFR 50.24.

In this important finding the IRB fails to document activities such as public consultation and disclosure of a clinical study under the requirements of 21 CFR 50.24. For review purposes under this section, these consultations are required to obtain from the public at large their position on whether subjects can be enrolled in a study without a written consent.

Findings Relating to IRB Review Process of Special Populations in Clinical Trials

(a) **Failure to ensure research involving children is in compliance with Part 50, subpart D, at the time of initial review of the research.** [21 CFR 56.109(h) and 21 CFR 50.50)

Let us examine the following:

The IRB failed to ensure that research involving children complied with the requirements listed in 21 CFR 50, subpart D—"Additional Safeguards for Children in Clinical Investigations." Specifically, the IRB approved Study Protocol [XX] on March 10, 2005. Even though this study allows enrollment of subjects as young as 12 years of age, there was no documentation in the IRB's files that the regulations involving safeguards for children were discussed or ensured.

Presently, there are more studies involving special populations such as children, the elderly, or mentally challenged patients. All IRBs should have documented requirements to safeguard the health, rights, and welfare of these populations.

An other example is the following:

The IRB failed to make determinations that research was in compliance with 21 CFR Part 50, Subpart D, in protocol [XX] among others. Subpart D requires the IRB to make a determination that the clinical investigation meets the requirements of one of these categories of research [50.51 (minimal risk), 50.52 (greater than minimal risk, but presenting the prospect of direct benefit), or 50.53 (greater than minimal risk and no prospect of direct benefit)]. San Juan IRB made determinations under Department of Health and Human Services regulations under Title 45, Part 46, Subpart D—Additional Protections for Children Involved as Subjects in Research in correspondence with investigators without referencing 21 CFR Subpart D. In addition, the determinations of protocol [XX] compliance with Title 45, Part 46, Subpart D are internally inconsistent.

IRBs have to comply with the provisions of 21 CFR 50 Part D, have to implement SOPs and must document adherence to those provisions in each relevant case.

Administrative Actions to IRBs
The following are administrative actions that the FDA may impose on a noncompliant IRB:

- Withhold approval of new studies that are conducted at the institution or reviewed by the IRB
- Direct that no new subjects be added to ongoing studies
- Terminate ongoing studies when doing so would not endanger the subjects

- Notify relevant state and federal regulatory agencies and other parties with direct interest in the FDA's action of the deficiencies in the operation of the IRB in instances when the apparent noncompliance creates a significant threat to the rights and welfare of human subjects

The FDA Commissioner can also begin proceedings to disqualify an IRB or the institution if the IRB has refused or repeatedly failed to comply with the FDA's IRB regulations (21 CFR Part 56) and the noncompliance adversely affects the rights or welfare of the human subjects in a clinical investigation. Disqualification may be initiated as follows:

(a) Whenever the IRB or the institution has failed to take adequate steps to correct the noncompliance stated in the letter sent by the agency under 56.120(a), and the Commissioner of Food and Drugs determines that this noncompliance may justify the disqualification of the IRB or of the parent institution, the Commissioner will institute proceedings in accordance with the requirements for a regulatory hearing set forth in part 16.

(b) The Commissioner may disqualify an IRB or the parent institution if the Commissioner determines that:

  (i) The IRB has refused or repeatedly failed to comply with any of the regulations set forth in this part, and

  (ii) The noncompliance adversely affects the rights or welfare of the human subjects in a clinical investigation.

(c) If the Commissioner determines that disqualification is appropriate, the Commissioner will issue an order that explains the basis for the determination and that prescribes any actions to be taken with regard to ongoing clinical research conducted under the review of the IRB. The Food and Drug Administration will send notice of the disqualification to the IRB and the parent institution. Other parties with a direct interest, such as sponsors and clinical investigators, may also be sent a notice of the disqualification. In addition, the agency may elect to publish a notice of its action in the *Federal Register*.

The consequences of an IRB's disqualification on the sponsor's development of a product are immense. The Food and Drug Administration will not approve an application for a research permit for a clinical investigation that is to be under the review of a disqualified IRB or that is to be conducted at a disqualified institution, and it may refuse to consider (in support of a marketing permit) the data from a clinical investigation that was reviewed by a disqualified IRB or conducted at a disqualified institution, unless the IRB or the parent institution is reinstated as provided in 56.123.

Reinstatement of a Disqualified IRB

An IRB or an institution may be reinstated if the Commissioner determines, upon an evaluation of a written submission from the IRB or institution that explains the corrective action that the institution or IRB plans to take, that the IRB or institution has provided adequate assurance that it will operate in compliance with the standards set forth in this part. Notification of reinstatement shall be provided to all persons notified under 56.121(c).

Conclusions on the Findings   It seems very obvious that the main finding here is that some IRBs and investigators are not properly trained to perform clinical trial activities in compliance with regulatory requirements. "Obliviousness" seems to be the perfect descriptive term for the fact that explicit requirements were not followed. Investigators as well as IRB members can misconstrue the requirements and innocently/unintentionally did not follow their own procedures. Clinical trials have become very complicated, to the extent that investigators become bewildered by the amount of data to be collected and perhaps by the new technology to be mastered. Unless guided (holding hands in the beginning if necessary) by a knowledgeable sponsor, they get lost in the complex protocol instructions and become noncompliant.

The most viable solution to this particular issue is to provide extensive training in clinical research for investigators, clinical trial personnel at the site, and IRB members by expert clinical research professionals. A clear effort to train investigators will provide high returns on investment as more quality data and better compliance are achieved.

CHAPTER 5

FRAUD AND MISCONDUCT IN CLINICAL RESEARCH

Clinical trial misconduct is not common. However, it may affect the public confidence in the clinical trial process. Monitoring has become an activity that requires extensive resources and is limited by the time constraints of a clinical trial. Monitoring is performed by comparison of data, not questioning the validity of the sources if they are consistent with the CRFs and the clinical trial protocol.

The sponsor has the responsibility of selecting the right investigator, utilizing a proven site feasibility process where many factors are taken into account for selection. Once the investigator sites are chosen, proper training and support should be provided to continuously assist the sites in the task of running a compliant study, enrolling the right patients, and capturing the right information.

Nevertheless, there is always the possibility that things do not go as planned.

Therefore, the FDA in its effort to ensure public safety also focuses on the possibility of **falsification of data**. Falsification or fraud is interpreted as purposely misleading the public and the FDA on the safety and efficacy of a therapeutic product. Everything revolves around data quality, integrity, and auditability. Research misconduct can be at any level of science, whereas the falsification of data can be found in the design and implementation of the clinical trial protocol, data capture, resolution and analysis, monitoring, and quality assurance. Falsification also means omission of data or commission of data. Acts of omission may be perpetrated purposely or unintentionally where specific data is not reported (e.g., underreporting of adverse events because either the investigator does not agree with the terminology or does not like that data). Omission of safety data may expose the subjects to a higher risk than expected. Acts of commission are defined as purposely altering data to make it look better (e.g., out of range laboratory values are reported by the investigator as clinically insignificant to override the classification as an adverse event). Another aspect of data falsification is the interpretation of results after analysis to downplay a serious issue (e.g., the number of cases with this serious adverse event is not different from the total number of cases observed in postmarketing surveillance for the same type of product in the general population—we are diluting the impact of the SAE).

What is the FDA position on research misconduct?

The FDA interprets clinical research misconduct as deliberate or repeated noncompliance with the regulations. Research misconduct does not include honest error or honest differences in opinion. At this point, it is important to make a clarification that the principal investigator is brought into a clinical trial to provide sponsors with a medical opinion on the safety and efficacy of an investigational product, and differences of opinions will exist: those are very important to annotate to be able to draw a final valid conclusion.

Data falsification is **fraud**, a felony, and further increases the risk of subjects participating in a study, and jeopardizes the reliability of the data. If the FDA or any other agency bases its conclusion on the safety and efficacy of a therapeutic product on false data, their mission of safeguarding the health of the people cannot be accomplished.

Fraud at the level of the clinical trial site can have a wide impact, since one investigator may be providing safety and efficacy data from multiple studies to many sponsors. Therefore, having a handful of fraudulent investigators may have a serious impact on the safety and efficacy of several marketed products. For example, one investigator may be involved in 91 applications for 47 different sponsors.

From FDA inspectional experience, we can ask the following:

- What type of data is falsified?
- How is data falsified?
- Why is data falsified?
- Who falsified the data?
- What can be done to detect fraud?
- How do we prevent fraud?

5.1   WHAT TYPE OF DATA IS FALSIFIED?

- Blood pressure
- Weight
- Biological specimens
- Physical and laboratory examinations
- Subject identities
- Drug accountability records
- EEG, EKG, and so on
- All clinical trial data can be falsified

For example, the FDA inspectors observed that there are leads to detect fraud in clinical research as follows:

- The investigator keeps stock files of EKGs.
- There are Identical duplicate prints of X rays with different names.
- Blank copies of lab reports are used to produce fake reports.

- An original lab report was never filed and these are multiple copies of one report under different names.
- The names of deceased persons are used.
- There are unopened boxes of investigational product that was reported as used.

Noncompliance issues may also arouse the suspicion of misconduct as follows:

- Dates were changed on EKGs to coincide with the proper visit in the protocol.
- The investigator used old EKG tracings for recent visits.
- Subjects may meet exclusion criteria but continued in the study to achieve enrollment objectives.
- Noncompliance is observed in the consenting process.
- Data collected in CRFs was not supported by the progress notes.

All these observations indicate that the investigator purposely misled the FDA in creating the data.

5.2   HOW IS DATA FALSIFIED?

Investigators resort to all kinds of manipulations with the intent to mislead.

Electrocardiograms

- The continuous strip run of one patient was torn in half to represent the run of another patient.
- The preprinted subject information on the EKG was purposely changed.
- Other EKGs were photocopied.

Blood Pressure Data

- BP data and date were changed as to the source to match the CRF and vice versa.
- BP values were fudged, overriding the source data, to represent the ideal patient sought in the protocol criteria. (The investigator may be under pressure to enroll any patient to meet an enrollment target.)

In the previous example, when the FDA inspector asked about the book perfect blood pressure values, the response he got is that the population is different from the U.S. population. Look for odd answers to direct questions!

Physical or Laboratory Examination Data

- The normality or abnormality of the result may only be checked in one box in the CRF without source documentation.
- Falsified lab reports are concocted to make patients meet inclusion criteria.

Biological Specimens

- Samples purported to come from a large number of individual subjects were actually derived from only a few different subjects.
- The investigator divided the samples to "produce" more patients.

Investigational Product

- Drug compliance records showed 100% compliance in taking test medication as recorded in CRFs.
- The reality was that the returned study drug was dumped (too much work to check for compliance, or just negligence).

5.3 WHY IS DATA FALSIFIED?

This is a complicated question. There may be many reasons; however, some of them could be:

- Greed, to make the most out of a trial
- Complete protocol enrollment because an agreement was signed
- Meet study targets to please the sponsor
- To earn academic or scientific merit (if not caught)
- Not enough time or loss of interest
- Staff turnover
- Not enough subjects
- For the "good of subject"
- Pressure to publish
- Obliviousness

5.4 WHO FALSIFIED THE DATA?

Basically, we should ask who will benefit from the falsification of data, and there we will have the answer.

The most conspicuous case was from Robert Fiddes, MD, who was found guilty of conspiracy to commit an offense against the United States, and guilty of making false statements in a matter within the jurisdiction of the FDA (18 USC 1001). He was sentenced to 15 months in jail, fined U.S. $800,000, and deported.

From the information provided by the FDA, he was supposed to enroll patients who tested positive for the presence of bacteria in the ear canal. Basically, he purchased the bacteria and sent samples to a lab for analysis as if they belonged to enrolled patients. In this case, unless we summon all the patients, from the data presented there was no indication that the patients did not exist. A whistleblower was the key to detect this case since he passed most inspections.

5.5   WHAT CAN BE DONE TO DETECT FRAUD?

It is not a simple task to detect fraud; however, leads should be investigated. We also have many new tools that were not readily available 20 years ago. If the sponsor suspects fraud, it may prompt the following action to gather evidence. For example, in a chronic bronchitis study, 84 of the subjects enrolled were required to produce positive sputum samples to qualify for study. The monitor reported that sputum samples were not collected as per the protocol (i.e., in the presence of the investigator). The FDA inspected and the sponsor audited to validate data. No direct evidence of a problem with specimen integrity was found. However, the sponsor was suspicious. Therefore, the sponsor performed DNA analysis on sputum and serum samples to put concerns to rest. The results of the analysis showed 35 of 84 sets of subject serum and sputum samples did not match, and 26 sputum samples were found to be derived from only 3 subjects. Therefore, subject identities had been altered: the same subject was enrolled more than once under two different names and subject numbers, and nonexistent subjects were created with other's samples.

In another case, a doctor fabricated laboratory data and eye exams for all subjects. He created data for subjects by using available results from different subjects in his office, and recycled subjects (three times) and invented data (EKG tracings, duplicate lab results). He also used 2-year-old EKG tracings. This was detected in an inspection. He was disqualified as an investigator.

In an older case, Dr. K. in 1987 submitted 85 cases of which only 15 were real subjects. He faked approximately 70 subjects' records and never used the test article—he used marketed products. By the way, he did not obtain informed consent. This investigator was also disqualified. He was also sentenced to 400 hours of community service and fined U.S. $30,000.

5.6   HOW DO WE PREVENT FRAUD?

Fraud is a possibility in any human activity. The sponsor of a clinical trial should take that possibility seriously, including it as part of the risk approach. The sponsor and the investigator can join efforts to prevent fraud in a constructive manner. The following are some approaches that may be employed:

- Clinical trial protocols should be less complex, to avoid placing needless requirements or unreasonable demands on the site.
- The study site should have the necessary resources and support to accomplish its tasks.
- Monitor sites closely and pay attention to complaints from site personnel.
- Minimize the use of enrollment incentives.

The monitor and/or the internal auditor should have a company set criteria to determine veracity of the data presented by the investigator. Some of the criteria may include the following:

- Understand the protocol and the investigational plan.
- Identify key parameters for the inclusion and exclusion criteria.
- Identify all source documents for data entered in the CRFs.
- Request all supporting evidence for critical data in the clinical trial (laboratory test results, X rays, CT scans, MRI scans, and other reports).
- Accept only originals as the source.
- Look for errors in data entry and for corrections.
- Request justification for each entry corrected to be supported by a valid source document.
- Challenge suspicious data.
- Record all observations in a monitoring report or audit report.
- If you consider that something is not right (gut feeling) try to find the inconsistency and document your findings.
- If something looks too good to be true, maybe it is. Review critical data again.

Serious misconduct can be detected if the monitor is prepared for the task. The following steps may increase the chances of detecting fraud:

- *Build Expertise.* The monitor should be prepared to understand the materials to be monitored, not only to produce a mere inventory during the visit. The monitor should be able to read any X rays to determine if the patient is male or female, compare EKGs between visits and patients, assess laboratory results as to data inconsistency, and compare laboratory tests.
- *Perform Data Quality Checks.* If there are missing dates, times, or other information in the CRF, before asking the investigator, check the source documents and cross-check with other site records.
- *Present the Possibility that the Data Is Not Source Verifiable.* Avoid confrontation with the investigator. Create a complete report, copying all data and documents that can make your case.
- *Sponsor's Responsibility.* The Sposnor should consider the monitor's concerns and address them.
- *Investigator's Responsibility.* Remind the Investigator of his/her responsibilities for the conduct of the study.
- *Expect Fraud as a Possibility.* Determine that the data and supporting information are not flawed in any way.
- *Interact Actively with the Site Staff.* Monitoring should be conducted periodically as deemed necessary to assure compliance. Be there as often as possible and be available to respond to any issue. Listen and read between the lines.

The FDA has summarized the complaints made by different parties, including sponsors of clinical trials, site personnel, patients, IRBs, and others. Those complaints against investigative sites are as follows (quantity of cases reported in parentheses):

- Failure to follow the protocol (70)
- Falsification (67)
- Informed consent issues (55)
- Failure to report adverse events (40)
- Qualifications of persons performing physicals (27)
- Inadequate records (25)
- Failure to get IRB approval or report changes in research (20)
- Failure to follow FDA regulations (13)
- Charging for the test article (9)
- Drug accountability (7)
- No active IND (7)
- Violations of GLP (7)
- Misleading advertisements (5)
- Blinding (3)
- No Form 1572 Submitted (2)
- Monitoring practices (2)
- IRB shopping (1)

Falsification of data is high up in the list of complaints against investigator sites. The FDA expects that the sponsor immediately reports misconduct that ranges from chronic noncompliance and refusal to comply to regulatory requirements to falsification of data, even before a site is terminated.

In summary, although fraud in clinical trials is not a common event, the sponsor should have the procedures implemented to provide the monitor with tools to detect falsification of data. Training monitors in all aspects of clinical trial monitoring, including misconduct, and providing them with effective support will allow the sponsor to be on top of all trial situations that may endanger the future of the development plan. Proactive measures, such as internal compliance inspections of critical sites, will allow sponsors to remain confident that a proper follow-up on studies was conducted.

SOME ANSWERS TO THE MOST PROBLEMATIC QUESTIONS IN COMPLIANCE

HOW CAN AN INVESTIGATOR SITE DEMONSTRATE THAT THE PROPER CONSENT PROCESS WAS FOLLOWED?

The site should have to implement fully compliant standard operating procedures for consenting subjects, where a detailed description of the process exists. Full continuous training should be provided to all site personnel involved in the consenting process and it should be documented. Quality assurance of the implemented procedure should exist to ensure that the process is followed for all clinical trials. The principal investigator should be involved at arm's length in the consenting of the subjects and controlling that the SOPs are followed.

HOW DOES ONE DEMONSTRATE THAT A SUBJECT UNDERSTOOD THE CONSENT INFORMATION?

Although the signature on the consent document should mean that the patient understood the investigational procedures, the question remains: did he/she?

Actually, there are many approaches an investigator can follow to convince him/herself that the subject really understood. One of them is administration of a quiz that the subject must respond to and pass before signing the consent. Another is having the subject describe what he/she understood with respect to the clinical trial procedures and his/her responsibilities and rights. Lastly, subjects are allowed enough time to read at their own pace. Investigators should make notes of all questions in writing and provide the answers also in writing.

Next, there is the issue of subjects who cannot consent for themselves but a legal representative signs the consent for the study and procedures on behalf of the patient. In that case, every effort should be documented to explain the investigational study to the subject and, if possible, also obtain his/her consent.

Clinical Trials Audit Preparation: A Guide for Good Clinical Practice (GCP) Inspections, by Vera Mihajlovic-Madzarevic
Copyright © 2010 John Wiley & Sons, Inc.

HOW DOES ONE DEMONSTRATE THAT ALL THE CLINICAL TRIAL PROCEDURES WERE FOLLOWED?

When the procedure involves drug accountability, physical examination, or clinical trial laboratory tests, it is more evident how to demonstrate that the procedures were followed. In the case of drug accountability, keeping a neat accountability log will demonstrate compliance. For physical examination, the investigator records all findings in the patient files. And for laboratory tests, the laboratory reports together with the sample collection logs are evidence that suffice to meet the requirement.

But what about the case, for example, where the patient should take study medication 1 hour before meals on an empty stomach and with 300 mL of water? This case is more complicated because the investigator or coordinators are not there to make notes of all the activities. In that case, the patient should make every effort to follow the procedure and keep a diary: if a deviation occurs such as forgetting to take a dose or not finishing the glass of water, these can be recorded.

In the case, for example, where the patient is to consume no more than 1 gram of fat per day during active treatment with study medication, it becomes more challenging to demonstrate that the patient followed the procedure. In this case, a simple food diary will allow the investigator to check compliance; however, remember that the patient can also cheat.

There should be two elements to demonstrate compliance to procedures: one is the intent of the investigator to ensure compliance, and the other is the effectiveness and reliability of the method selected. Bottom line, there is a limit how far we can go to demonstrate adherence to procedures, and we can go as far as humanly possible.

HOW DOES ONE DEMONSTRATE PRINCIPAL INVESTIGATOR PERSONAL INVOLVEMENT IN THE SUPERVISION OF CLINICAL TRIAL ACTIVITIES?

The investigator site should have procedures for delegation of responsibilities as well as supervision and accountability. The investigator should account for, with written documentation, his/her personal involvement in the medical decisions for patients or direct supervision of qualified delegates. Detailed minutes of meetings conducted periodically to discuss the clinical trial with clinical trial personnel may provide such evidence.

WHY FOLLOW STANDARD OPERATING PROCEDURES IN CLINICAL TRIALS?

SOPs are going to be inspected together with all clinical trial documents. The audited SOPs should be the effective versions at the time of the study. SOPs provide the party (sponsor, investigator, or IRB) with compliant procedures to avoid noncompliance issues. Following the SOP manual will allow you to remain on track with what is required from you for a particular activity (remember that the SOPs have to be properly written and compliant themselves).

GUIDANCE FOR INDUSTRY*—E6 GOOD CLINICAL PRACTICE: CONSOLIDATED GUIDANCE

---

*This guidance was developed within the Expert Working Group (Efficacy) of the International Conference on Harmonisation of Technical Requirements for Registration of Pharmaceuticals for Human Use (ICH) and has been subject to consultation by the regulatory parties, in accordance with the ICH process. This document has been endorsed by the ICH Steering Committee at *Step 4* of the ICH process, April 1996. At *Step 4* of the process, the final draft is recommended for adoption to the regulatory bodies of the European Union, Japan, and the United States. This guidance was published in the *Federal Register* on May 9, 1997 (62 FR 25692) and is applicable to drug and biological products. This guidance represents the FDA's current thinking on good clinical practices. It does not create or confer any rights for or on any person and does not operate to bind the FDA or the public. An alternative approach may be used if such approach satisfies the requirements of the applicable statute, regulations, or both.

Clinical Trials Audit Preparation: A Guide for Good Clinical Practice (GCP) Inspections, by Vera Mihajlovic-Madzarevic
Copyright © 2010 John Wiley & Sons, Inc.

INTRODUCTION

Good clinical practice (GCP) is an international ethical and scientific quality standard for designing, conducting, recording, and reporting trials that involve the participation of human subjects. Compliance with this standard provides public assurance that the rights, safety, and well-being of trial subjects are protected, consistent with the principles that have their origin in the Declaration of Helsinki, and that the clinical trial data are credible.

The objective of this ICH GCP guidance is to provide a unified standard for the European Union (EU), Japan, and the United States to facilitate the mutual acceptance of clinical data by the regulatory authorities in these jurisdictions.

The guidance was developed with consideration of the current good clinical practices of the European Union, Japan, and the United States, as well as those of Australia, Canada, the Nordic countries, and the World Health Organization (WHO).

This guidance should be followed when generating clinical trial data that are intended to be submitted to regulatory authorities.

The principles established in this guidance may also be applied to other clinical investigations that may have an impact on the safety and well-being of human subjects.

1. GLOSSARY

1.1 Adverse Drug Reaction (ADR): In the preapproval clinical experience with a new medicinal product or its new usages, particularly as the therapeutic dose(s) may not be established, all noxious and unintended responses to a medicinal product related to any dose should be considered adverse drug reactions. The phrase "responses to a medicinal product" means that a causal relationship between a medicinal product and an adverse event is at least a reasonable possibility, i.e., the relationship cannot be ruled out.

Regarding marketed medicinal products: A response to a drug that is noxious and unintended and that occurs at doses normally used in man for prophylaxis, diagnosis, or therapy of diseases or for modification of physiological function (see the ICH guidance for Clinical Safety Data Management: Definitions and Standards for Expedited Reporting).

1.2   Adverse Event (AE): An AE is any untoward medical occurrence in a patient or clinical investigation subject administered a pharmaceutical product and that does not necessarily have a causal relationship with this treatment. An AE can therefore be any unfavorable and unintended sign (including an abnormal laboratory finding), symptom, or disease temporally associated with the use of a medicinal (investigational) product, whether or not related to the medicinal (investigational) product (see the ICH guidance for Clinical Safety Data Management: Definitions and Standards for Expedited Reporting).

1.3   Amendment (to the Protocol): See Protocol Amendment.

1.4   Applicable Regulatory Requirement(s): Any law(s) and regulation(s) addressing the conduct of clinical trials of investigational products of the jurisdiction where trial is conducted.

1.5   Approval (in Relation to Institutional Review Boards (IRBs)): The affirmative decision of the IRB that the clinical trial has been reviewed and may be conducted at the institution site within the constraints set forth by the IRB, the institution, good clinical practice (GCP), and the applicable regulatory requirements.

1.6   Audit: A systematic and independent examination of trial-related activities and documents to determine whether the evaluated trial-related activities were conducted, and the data were recorded, analyzed, and accurately reported according to the protocol, sponsor's standard operating procedures (SOPs), good clinical practice (GCP), and the applicable regulatory requirement(s).

1.7   Audit Certificate: A declaration of confirmation by the auditor that an audit has taken place.

1.8   Audit Report: A written evaluation by the sponsor's auditor of the results of the audit.

1.9   Audit Trail: Documentation that allows reconstruction of the course of events.

1.10 Blinding/Masking: A procedure in which one or more parties to the trial are kept unaware of the treatment assignment(s). Single blinding usually refers to the subject(s) being unaware, and double blinding usually refers to the subject(s), investigator(s), monitor, and, in some cases, data analyst(s) being unaware of the treatment assignment(s).

1.11 Case Report Form (CRF): A printed, optical, or electronic document designed to record all of the protocol-required information to be reported to the sponsor on each trial subject.

1.12 Clinical Trial/Study: Any investigation in human subjects intended to discover or verify the clinical, pharmacological, and/or other pharmacodynamic effects of an investigational product(s), and/or to identify any adverse reactions to an investigational product(s), and/or to study absorption, distribution, metabolism, and excretion of an investigational product(s) with the object of ascertaining its safety and/or efficacy. The terms clinical trial and clinical study are synonymous.

1.13 Clinical Trial/Study Report: A written description of a trial/study of any therapeutic, prophylactic, or diagnostic agent conducted in human subjects, in which the clinical and statistical description, presentations, and analyses are fully integrated into a single report (see the ICH Guidance for Structure and Content of Clinical Study Reports).

1.14 Comparator (Product): An investigational or marketed product (i.e., active control), or placebo, used as a reference in a clinical trial.

1.15 Compliance (in Relation to Trials): Adherence to all the trial-related requirements, good clinical practice (GCP) requirements, and the applicable regulatory requirements.

1.16 Confidentiality: Prevention of disclosure, to other than authorized individuals, of a sponsor's proprietary information or of a subject's identity.

1.17 Contract: A written, dated, and signed agreement between two or more involved parties that sets out any arrangements on delegation and distribution of tasks and obligations and, if appropriate, on financial matters. The protocol may serve as the basis of a contract.

1.18 Coordinating Committee: A committee that a sponsor may organize to coordinate the conduct of a multicenter trial.

1.19 Coordinating Investigator: An investigator assigned the responsibility for the coordination of investigators at different centers participating in a multicenter trial.

1.20 Contract Research Organization (CRO): A person or an organization (commercial, academic, or other) contracted by the sponsor to perform one or more of a sponsor's trial-related duties and functions.

1.21 Direct Access: Permission to examine, analyze, verify, and reproduce any records and reports that are important to evaluation of a clinical trial. Any party (e.g., domestic and foreign regulatory authorities, sponsors, monitors, and auditors) with direct access should take all reasonable precautions within the constraints of the applicable regulatory requirement(s) to maintain the confidentiality of subjects' identities and sponsor's proprietary information.

1.22 Documentation: All records, in any form (including, but not limited to, written, electronic, magnetic, and optical records; and scans, x-rays, and electrocardiograms) that describe or record the methods, conduct, and/or results of a trial, the factors affecting a trial, and the actions taken.

1.23 Essential Documents: Documents that individually and collectively permit evaluation of the conduct of a study and the quality of the data produced (see section 8. "Essential Documents for the Conduct of a Clinical Trial").

1.24 Good Clinical Practice (GCP): A standard for the design, conduct, performance, monitoring, auditing, recording, analyses, and reporting of clinical trials that provides assurance that the data and reported results are credible and accurate, and that the rights, integrity, and confidentiality of trial subjects are protected.

1.25 Independent Data Monitoring Committee (IDMC) (Data and Safety Monitoring Board, Monitoring Committee, Data Monitoring Committee): An independent data monitoring committee that may be established by the sponsor to assess at intervals the progress of a clinical trial, the safety data, and the critical efficacy endpoints, and to recommend to the sponsor whether to continue, modify, or stop a trial.

1.26 Impartial Witness: A person, who is independent of the trial, who cannot be unfairly influenced by people involved with the trial, who attends the informed consent process if the subject or the subject's legally acceptable representative cannot read, and who reads the informed consent form and any other written information supplied to the subject.

1.27 Independent Ethics Committee (IEC): An independent body (a review board or a committee, institutional, regional, national, or supranational), constituted of medical/scientific professionals and nonmedical/nonscientific members, whose responsibility it is to ensure the protection of the rights, safety, and well-being of human subjects involved in a trial and to provide public assurance of that protection, by, among other things, reviewing and approving/providing favorable opinion on the trial protocol, the suitability of the investigator(s), facilities, and the methods and material to be used in obtaining and documenting informed consent of the trial subjects.

The legal status, composition, function, operations, and regulatory requirements pertaining to Independent Ethics Committees may differ among countries, but should allow the Independent Ethics Committee to act in agreement with GCP as described in this guidance.

1.28 Informed Consent: A process by which a subject voluntarily confirms his or her willingness to participate in a particular trial, after having been informed of all aspects of the trial that are relevant to the subject's decision to participate. Informed consent is documented by means of a written, signed, and dated informed consent form.

1.29 Inspection: The act by a regulatory authority(ies) of conducting an official review of documents, facilities, records, and any other resources that are deemed by the authority(ies) to be related to the clinical trial and that may be located at the site of the trial, at the sponsor's and/or contract research organization's (CROs) facilities, or at other establishments deemed appropriate by the regulatory authority(ies).

1.30 Institution (Medical): Any public or private entity or agency or medical or dental facility where clinical trials are conducted.

1.31 Institutional Review Board (IRB): An independent body constituted of medical, scientific, and nonscientific members, whose responsibility it is to ensure the protection of the rights, safety, and well-being of human subjects involved in a trial by, among other things, reviewing, approving, and providing continuing review of trials, of protocols and amendments, and of the methods and material to be used in obtaining and documenting informed consent of the trial subjects.

1.32 Interim Clinical Trial/Study Report: A report of intermediate results and their evaluation based on analyses performed during the course of a trial.

1.33 Investigational Product: A pharmaceutical form of an active ingredient or placebo being tested or used as a reference in a clinical trial, including a product with a marketing authorization when used or assembled (formulated or packaged) in a way different from the approved form, or when used for an unapproved indication, or when used to gain further information about an approved use.

1.34 Investigator: A person responsible for the conduct of the clinical trial at a trial site. If a trial is conducted by a team of individuals at a trial site, the investigator is the responsible leader of the team and may be called the principal investigator. See also Subinvestigator.

1.35 Investigator/Institution: An expression meaning "the investigator and/or institution, where required by the applicable regulatory requirements."

1.36 Investigator's Brochure: A compilation of the clinical and nonclinical data on the investigational product(s) that is relevant to the study of the investigational product(s) in human subjects (see section 7. "Investigator's Brochure").

1.37 Legally Acceptable Representative: An individual or juridical or other body authorized under applicable law to consent, on behalf of a prospective subject, to the subject's participation in the clinical trial.

1.38 Monitoring: The act of overseeing the progress of a clinical trial, and of ensuring that it is conducted, recorded, and reported in accordance with the protocol, standard operating procedures (SOPs), GCP, and the applicable regulatory requirement(s).

1.39 Monitoring Report: A written report from the monitor to the sponsor after each site visit and/or other trial-related communication according to the sponsor's SOPs.

1.40 Multicenter Trial: A clinical trial conducted according to a single protocol but at more than one site, and, therefore, carried out by more than one investigator.

1.41 Nonclinical Study: Biomedical studies not performed on human subjects.

1.42 Opinion (in Relation to Independent Ethics Committee): The judgment and/or the advice provided by an Independent Ethics Committee (IEC).

1.43 Original Medical Record: See Source Documents.

1.44 Protocol: A document that describes the objective(s), design, methodology, statistical considerations, and organization of a trial. The protocol usually also gives the background and rationale for the trial, but these could be provided in other protocol referenced documents. Throughout the ICH GCP Guidance, the term protocol refers to protocol and protocol amendments.

1.45 Protocol Amendment: A written description of a change(s) to or formal clarification of a protocol.

1.46 Quality Assurance (QA): All those planned and systematic actions that are established to ensure that the trial is performed and the data are generated, documented (recorded), and reported in compliance with GCP and the applicable regulatory requirement(s).

1.47 Quality Control (QC): The operational techniques and activities undertaken within the quality assurance system to verify that the requirements for quality of the trial-related activities have been fulfilled.

1.48 Randomization: The process of assigning trial subjects to treatment or control groups using an element of chance to determine the assignments in order to reduce bias.

1.49 Regulatory Authorities: Bodies having the power to regulate. In the ICH GCP guidance, the expression "Regulatory Authorities" includes the authorities that review submitted clinical data and those that conduct inspections (see section 1.29). These bodies are sometimes referred to as competent authorities.

1.50 Serious Adverse Event (SAE) or Serious Adverse Drug Reaction (Serious ADR): Any untoward medical occurrence that at any dose:

- Results in death,
- Is life-threatening,
- Requires inpatient hospitalization or prolongation of existing hospitalization,
- Results in persistent or significant disability/incapacity, or
- Is a congenital anomaly/birth defect.

(See the ICH guidance for Clinical Safety Data Management: Definitions and Standards for Expedited Reporting.)

1.51 Source Data: All information in original records and certified copies of original records of clinical findings, observations, or other activities in a clinical trial necessary for the reconstruction and evaluation of the trial. Source data are contained in source documents (original records or certified copies).

1.52 Source Documents: Original documents, data, and records (e.g., hospital records, clinical and office charts, laboratory notes, memoranda, subjects' diaries or evaluation checklists, pharmacy dispensing records, recorded data from automated instruments, copies or transcriptions certified after verification as being accurate and complete, microfiches, photographic negatives, microfilm or magnetic media, x-rays, subject files, and records kept at the pharmacy, at the laboratories, and at medico-technical departments involved in the clinical trial).

1.53 Sponsor: An individual, company, institution, or organization that takes responsibility for the initiation, management, and/or financing of a clinical trial.

1.54 Sponsor-Investigator: An individual who both initiates and conducts, alone or with others, a clinical trial, and under whose immediate direction the investigational product is administered to, dispensed to, or used by a subject. The term does not include any person other than an individual (e.g., it does not include a corporation or an agency). The obligations of a sponsor-investigator include both those of a sponsor and those of an investigator.

1.55 Standard Operating Procedures (SOPs): Detailed, written instructions to achieve uniformity of the performance of a specific function.

1.56 Subinvestigator: Any individual member of the clinical trial team designated and supervised by the investigator at a trial site to perform critical trial-related procedures and/or to make important trial-related decisions (e.g., associates, residents, research fellows). See also Investigator.

1.57 Subject/Trial Subject: An individual who participates in a clinical trial, either as a recipient of the investigational product(s) or as a control.

1.58 Subject Identification Code: A unique identifier assigned by the investigator to each trial subject to protect the subject's identity and used in lieu of the subject's name when the investigator reports adverse events and/or other trial-related data.

1.59 Trial Site: The location(s) where trial-related activities are actually conducted.

1.60 Unexpected Adverse Drug Reaction: An adverse reaction, the nature or severity of which is not consistent with the applicable product information (e.g., Investigator's Brochure for an unapproved investigational product or package insert/summary of product characteristics for an approved product). (See the ICH Guidance for Clinical Safety Data Management: Definitions and Standards for Expedited Reporting.)

1.61 Vulnerable Subjects: Individuals whose willingness to volunteer in a clinical trial may be unduly influenced by the expectation, whether justified or not, of benefits associated with participation, or of a retaliatory response from senior members of a hierarchy in case of refusal to participate. Examples are members of a group with a hierarchical structure, such as medical, pharmacy, dental, and nursing students, subordinate hospital and laboratory personnel, employees of the pharmaceutical industry, members of the armed forces, and persons kept in detention. Other vulnerable subjects include patients with incurable diseases, persons in nursing homes, unemployed or impoverished persons, patients in emergency situations, ethnic minority groups, homeless persons, nomads, refugees, minors, and those incapable of giving consent.

1.62 Well-being (of the Trial Subjects): The physical and mental integrity of the subjects participating in a clinical trial.

2. THE PRINCIPLES OF ICH GCP

2.1 Clinical trials should be conducted in accordance with the ethical principles that have their origin in the Declaration of Helsinki, and that are consistent with GCP and the applicable regulatory requirement(s).

2.2 Before a trial is initiated, foreseeable risks and inconveniences should be weighed against the anticipated benefit for the individual trial subject and society. A trial should be initiated and continued only if the anticipated benefits justify the risks.

2.3 The rights, safety, and well-being of the trial subjects are the most important considerations and should prevail over interests of science and society.

2.4 The available nonclinical and clinical information on an investigational product should be adequate to support the proposed clinical trial.

2.5 Clinical trials should be scientifically sound, and described in a clear, detailed protocol.

2.6 A trial should be conducted in compliance with the protocol that has received prior institutional review board (IRB)/independent ethics committee (IEC) approval/favorable opinion.

2.7 The medical care given to, and medical decisions made on behalf of, subjects should always be the responsibility of a qualified physician or, when appropriate, of a qualified dentist.

2.8 Each individual involved in conducting a trial should be qualified by education, training, and experience to perform his or her respective task(s).

2.9 Freely given informed consent should be obtained from every subject prior to clinical trial participation.

2.10 All clinical trial information should be recorded, handled, and stored in a way that allows its accurate reporting, interpretation, and verification.

2.11 The confidentiality of records that could identify subjects should be protected, respecting the privacy and confidentiality rules in accordance with the applicable regulatory requirement(s).

2.12 Investigational products should be manufactured, handled, and stored in accordance with applicable good manufacturing practice (GMP). They should be used in accordance with the approved protocol.

2.13 Systems with procedures that assure the quality of every aspect of the trial should be implemented.

3. INSTITUTIONAL REVIEW BOARD/INDEPENDENT ETHICS COMMITTEE (IRB/IEC)

3.1 Responsibilities

3.1.1 An IRB/IEC should safeguard the rights, safety, and well-being of all trial subjects. Special attention should be paid to trials that may include vulnerable subjects.

3.1.2 The IRB/IEC should obtain the following documents:
Trial protocol(s)/amendment(s), written informed consent form(s) and consent form updates that the investigator proposes for use in the trial, subject recruitment procedures (e.g., advertisements), written information to be provided to subjects, Investigator's Brochure (IB), available safety information, information about payments and compensation available to subjects, the investigator's current curriculum vitae and/or other documentation evidencing qualifications, and any other documents that the IRB/IEC may require to fulfil its responsibilities.

The IRB/IEC should review a proposed clinical trial within a reasonable time and document its views in writing, clearly identifying the trial, the documents reviewed, and the dates for the following:

- Approval/favorable opinion;
- Modifications required prior to its approval/favorable opinion;
- Disapproval/negative opinion; and
- Termination/suspension of any prior approval/favorable opinion.

3.1.3 The IRB/IEC should consider the qualifications of the investigator for the proposed trial, as documented by a current curriculum vitae and/or by any other relevant documentation the IRB/IEC requests.

3.1.4 The IRB/IEC should conduct continuing review of each ongoing trial at intervals appropriate to the degree of risk to human subjects, but at least once per year.

3.1.5 The IRB/IEC may request more information than is outlined in paragraph 4.8.10 be given to subjects when, in the judgment of the IRB/IEC, the additional information would add meaningfully to the protection of the rights, safety, and/or well-being of the subjects.

3.1.6 When a nontherapeutic trial is to be carried out with the consent of the subject's legally acceptable representative (see sections 4.8.12, 4.8.14), the IRB/IEC should determine that the proposed protocol and/or other document(s) adequately addresses relevant ethical concerns and meets applicable regulatory requirements for such trials.

3.1.7 Where the protocol indicates that prior consent of the trial subject or the subject's legally acceptable representative is not possible (see section 4.8.15), the IRB/IEC should determine that the proposed protocol and/or other document(s) adequately addresses relevant ethical concerns and meets applicable regulatory requirements for such trials (i.e., in emergency situations).

3.1.8 The IRB/IEC should review both the amount and method of payment to subjects to assure that neither presents problems of coercion or undue influence on the trial subjects. Payments to a subject should be prorated and not wholly contingent on completion of the trial by the subject.

3.1.9 The IRB/IEC should ensure that information regarding payment to subjects, including the methods, amounts, and schedule of payment to trial subjects, is set forth in the written informed consent form and any other written information to be provided to subjects. The way payment will be prorated should be specified.

3.2 Composition, Functions, and Operations

3.2.1 The IRB/IEC should consist of a reasonable number of members, who collectively have the qualifications and experience to review and evaluate the science, medical aspects, and ethics of the proposed trial. It is recommended that the IRB/IEC should include:

(a) At least five members.

(b) At least one member whose primary area of interest is in a nonscientific area.

(c) At least one member who is independent of the institution/trial site.

Only those IRB/IEC members who are independent of the investigator and the sponsor of the trial should vote/provide opinion on a trial-related matter.

A list of IRB/IEC members and their qualifications should be maintained.

3.2.2 The IRB/IEC should perform its functions according to written operating procedures, should maintain written records of its activities and minutes of its meetings, and should comply with GCP and with the applicable regulatory requirement(s).

3.2.3 An IRB/IEC should make its decisions at announced meetings at which at least a quorum, as stipulated in its written operating procedures, is present.

3.2.4 Only members who participate in the IRB/IEC review and discussion should vote/provide their opinion and/or advise.

3.2.5 The investigator may provide information on any aspect of the trial, but should not participate in the deliberations of the IRB/IEC or in the vote/opinion of the IRB/IEC.

3.2.6 An IRB/IEC may invite nonmembers with expertise in special areas for assistance.

3.3 Procedures

The IRB/IEC should establish, document in writing, and follow its procedures, which should include:

3.3.1 Determining its composition (names and qualifications of the members) and the authority under which it is established.

3.3.2 Scheduling, notifying its members of, and conducting its meetings.

3.3.3 Conducting initial and continuing review of trials.

3.3.4 Determining the frequency of continuing review, as appropriate.

3.3.5 Providing, according to the applicable regulatory requirements, expedited review and approval/favorable opinion of minor change(s) in ongoing trials that have the approval/favorable opinion of the IRB/IEC.

3.3.6 Specifying that no subject should be admitted to a trial before the IRB/IEC issues its written approval/favorable opinion of the trial.

3.3.7 Specifying that no deviations from, or changes of, the protocol should be initiated without prior written IRB/IEC approval/favorable opinion of an appropriate amendment, except when necessary to eliminate immediate hazards to the subjects or when the change(s) involves only logistical or administrative aspects of the trial (e.g., change of monitor(s), telephone number(s)) (see section 4.5.2).

3.3.8 Specifying that the investigator should promptly report to the IRB/IEC:

(a) Deviations from, or changes of, the protocol to eliminate immediate hazards to the trial subjects (see sections 3.3.7, 4.5.2, 4.5.4).

(b) Changes increasing the risk to subjects and/or affecting significantly the conduct of the trial (see section 4.10.2).

(c) All adverse drug reactions (ADRs) that are both serious and unexpected.

(d) New information that may affect adversely the safety of the subjects or the conduct of the trial.

3.3.9 Ensuring that the IRB/IEC promptly notify in writing the investigator/institution concerning:

(a) Its trial-related decisions/opinions.

(b) The reasons for its decisions/opinions.

(c) Procedures for appeal of its decisions/opinions.

3.4 Records

The IRB/IEC should retain all relevant records (e.g., written procedures, membership lists, lists of occupations/affiliations of members, submitted documents, minutes of meetings, and correspondence) for a period of at least 3 years after completion of the trial and make them available upon request from the regulatory authority(ies).

The IRB/IEC may be asked by investigators, sponsors, or regulatory authorities to provide copies of its written procedures and membership lists.

4. INVESTIGATOR

4.1 Investigator's Qualifications and Agreements

4.1.1 The investigator(s) should be qualified by education, training, and experience to assume responsibility for the proper conduct of the trial, should meet all the qualifications specified by the applicable regulatory requirement(s), and should provide evidence of such qualifications through up-to-date curriculum vitae and/or other relevant documentation requested by the sponsor, the IRB/IEC, and/or the regulatory authority(ies).

4.1.2 The investigator should be thoroughly familiar with the appropriate use of the investigational product(s), as described in the protocol, in the current Investigator's Brochure, in the product information, and in other information sources provided by the sponsor.

4.1.3 The investigator should be aware of, and should comply with, GCP and the applicable regulatory requirements.

4.1.4 The investigator/institution should permit monitoring and auditing by the sponsor, and inspection by the appropriate regulatory authority(ies).

4.1.5   The investigator should maintain a list of appropriately qualified persons to whom the investigator has delegated significant trial-related duties.

4.2   Adequate Resources

4.2.1   The investigator should be able to demonstrate (e.g., based on retrospective data) a potential for recruiting the required number of suitable subjects within the agreed recruitment period.

4.2.2   The investigator should have sufficient time to properly conduct and complete the trial within the agreed trial period.

4.2.3   The investigator should have available an adequate number of qualified staff and adequate facilities for the foreseen duration of the trial to conduct the trial properly and safely.

4.2.4   The investigator should ensure that all persons assisting with the trial are adequately informed about the protocol, the investigational product(s), and their trial-related duties and functions.

4.3   Medical Care of Trial Subjects

4.3.1   A qualified physician (or dentist, when appropriate), who is an investigator or a subinvestigator for the trial, should be responsible for all trial-related medical (or dental) decisions.

4.3.2   During and following a subject's participation in a trial, the investigator/institution should ensure that adequate medical care is provided to a subject for any adverse events, including clinically significant laboratory values, related to the trial. The investigator/institution should inform a subject when medical care is needed for intercurrent illness(es) of which the investigator becomes aware.

4.3.3   It is recommended that the investigator inform the subject's primary physician about the subject's participation in the trial if the subject has a primary physician and if the subject agrees to the primary physician being informed.

4.3.4   Although a subject is not obliged to give his/her reason(s) for withdrawing prematurely from a trial, the investigator should make a reasonable effort to ascertain the reason(s), while fully respecting the subject's rights.

4.4   Communication with IRB/IEC

4.4.1   Before initiating a trial, the investigator/institution should have written and dated approval/favorable opinion from the IRB/IEC for the trial protocol, written informed consent form, consent form updates, subject recruitment procedures (e.g., advertisements), and any other written information to be provided to subjects.

4.4.2   As part of the investigator's/institution's written application to the IRB/IEC, the investigator/institution should provide the IRB/IEC with a current copy of the Investigator's Brochure. If the Investigator's Brochure is updated during the trial, the investigator/institution should supply a copy of the updated Investigator's Brochure to the IRB/IEC.

4.4.3   During the trial the investigator/institution should provide to the IRB/IEC all documents subject to its review.

4.5 Compliance with Protocol

4.5.1 The investigator/institution should conduct the trial in compliance with the protocol agreed to by the sponsor and, if required, by the regulatory authority(ies), and which was given approval/favorable opinion by the IRB/IEC. The investigator/institution and the sponsor should sign the protocol, or an alternative contract, to confirm their agreement.

4.5.2 The investigator should not implement any deviation from, or changes of, the protocol without agreement by the sponsor and prior review and documented approval/favorable opinion from the IRB/IEC of an amendment, except where necessary to eliminate an immediate hazard(s) to trial subjects, or when the change(s) involves only logistical or administrative aspects of the trial (e.g., change of monitor(s), change of telephone number(s)).

4.5.3 The investigator, or person designated by the investigator, should document and explain any deviation from the approved protocol.

4.5.4 The investigator may implement a deviation from, or a change in, the protocol to eliminate an immediate hazard(s) to trial subjects without prior IRB/IEC approval/favorable opinion. As soon as possible, the implemented deviation or change, the reasons for it, and, if appropriate, the proposed protocol amendment(s) should be submitted:

    (a) To the IRB/IEC for review and approval/favorable opinion;

    (b) To the sponsor for agreement and, if required;

    (c) To the regulatory authority(ies).

4.6 Investigational Product(s)

4.6.1 Responsibility for investigational product(s) accountability at the trial site(s) rests with the investigator/institution.

4.6.2 Where allowed/required, the investigator/institution may/should assign some or all of the investigator's/institution's duties for investigational product(s) accountability at the trial site(s) to an appropriate pharmacist or another appropriate individual who is under the supervision of the investigator/institution.

4.6.3 The investigator/institution and/or a pharmacist or other appropriate individual, who is designated by the investigator/institution, should maintain records of the product's delivery to the trial site, the inventory at the site, the use by each subject, and the return to the sponsor or alternative disposition of unused product(s). These records should include dates, quantities, batch/serial numbers, expiration dates (if applicable), and the unique code numbers assigned to the investigational product(s) and trial subjects. Investigators should maintain records that document adequately that the subjects were provided the doses specified by the protocol and reconcile all investigational product(s) received from the sponsor.

4.6.4 The investigational product(s) should be stored as specified by the sponsor (see sections 5.13.2 and 5.14.3) and in accordance with applicable regulatory requirement(s).

4.6.5 The investigator should ensure that the investigational product(s) are used only in accordance with the approved protocol.

4.6.6 The investigator, or a person designated by the investigator/institution, should explain the correct use of the investigational product(s) to each subject and should check, at intervals appropriate for the trial, that each subject is following the instructions properly.

4.7 Randomization Procedures and Unblinding

The investigator should follow the trial's randomization procedures, if any, and should ensure that the code is broken only in accordance with the protocol. If the trial is blinded, the investigator should promptly document and explain to the sponsor any premature unblinding (e.g., accidental unblinding, unblinding due to a serious adverse event) of the investigational product(s).

4.8 Informed Consent of Trial Subjects

4.8.1 In obtaining and documenting informed consent, the investigator should comply with the applicable regulatory requirement(s), and should adhere to GCP and to the ethical principles that have their origin in the Declaration of Helsinki. Prior to the beginning of the trial, the investigator should have the IRB/IEC's written approval/favorable opinion of the written informed consent form and any other written information to be provided to subjects.

4.8.2 The written informed consent form and any other written information to be provided to subjects should be revised whenever important new information becomes available that may be relevant to the subject's consent. Any revised written informed consent form, and written information should receive the IRB/IEC's approval/favorable opinion in advance of use. The subject or the subject's legally acceptable representative should be informed in a timely manner if new information becomes available that may be relevant to the subject's willingness to continue participation in the trial. The communication of this information should be documented.

4.8.3 Neither the investigator, nor the trial staff, should coerce or unduly influence a subject to participate or to continue to participate in a trial.

4.8.4 None of the oral and written information concerning the trial, including the written informed consent form, should contain any language that causes the subject or the subject's legally acceptable representative to waive or to appear to waive any legal rights, or that releases or appears to release the investigator, the institution, the sponsor, or their agents from liability for negligence.

4.8.5 The investigator, or a person designated by the investigator, should fully inform the subject or, if the subject is unable to provide informed consent, the subject's legally acceptable representative, of all pertinent aspects of the trial including the written information given approval/favorable opinion by the IRB/IEC.

4.8.6 The language used in the oral and written information about the trial, including the written informed consent form, should be as nontechnical as practical and should be understandable to the subject or the subject's legally acceptable representative and the impartial witness, where applicable.

4.8.7 Before informed consent may be obtained, the investigator, or a person designated by the investigator, should provide the subject or the subject's legally acceptable representative ample time and opportunity to inquire about details of the trial and to decide whether or not to participate in the trial. All questions about the trial should be answered to the satisfaction of the subject or the subject's legally acceptable representative.

4.8.8 Prior to a subject's participation in the trial, the written informed consent form should be signed and personally dated by the subject or by the subject's legally acceptable representative, and by the person who conducted the informed consent discussion.

4.8.9 If a subject is unable to read or if a legally acceptable representative is unable to read, an impartial witness should be present during the entire informed consent discussion. After the written informed consent form and any other written information to be provided to subjects is read and explained to the subject or the subject's legally acceptable representative, and after the subject or the subject's legally acceptable representative has orally consented to the subject's participation in the trial, and, if capable of doing so, has signed and personally dated the informed consent form, the witness should sign and personally date the consent form. By signing the consent form, the witness attests that the information in the consent form and any other written information was accurately explained to, and apparently understood by, the subject or the subject's legally acceptable representative, and that informed consent was freely given by the subject or the subject's legally acceptable representative.

4.8.10 Both the informed consent discussion and the written informed consent form and any other written information to be provided to subjects should include explanations of the following:

(a) That the trial involves research.

(b) The purpose of the trial.

(c) The trial treatment(s) and the probability for random assignment to each treatment.

(d) The trial procedures to be followed, including all invasive procedures.

(e) The subject's responsibilities.

(f) Those aspects of the trial that are experimental.

(g) The reasonably foreseeable risks or inconveniences to the subject and, when applicable, to an embryo, fetus, or nursing infant.

(h) The reasonably expected benefits. When there is no intended clinical benefit to the subject, the subject should be made aware of this.

(i) The alternative procedure(s) or course(s) of treatment that may be available to the subject, and their important potential benefits and risks.

(j) The compensation and/or treatment available to the subject in the event of trial-related injury.

(k) The anticipated prorated payment, if any, to the subject for participating in the trial.

(l) The anticipated expenses, if any, to the subject for participating in the trial.

(m) That the subject's participation in the trial is voluntary and that the subject may refuse to participate or withdraw from the trial, at any time, without penalty or loss of benefits to which the subject is otherwise entitled.

(n) That the monitor(s), the auditor(s), the IRB/IEC, and the regulatory authority(ies) will be granted direct access to the subject's original medical records for verification of clinical trial procedures and/or data, without violating the confidentiality of the subject, to the extent permitted by the applicable laws and regulations and that, by signing a written informed consent form, the subject or the subject's legally acceptable representative is authorizing such access.

(o) That records identifying the subject will be kept confidential and, to the extent permitted by the applicable laws and/or regulations, will not be made publicly available. If the results of the trial are published, the subject's identity will remain confidential.

(p) That the subject or the subject's legally acceptable representative will be informed in a timely manner if information becomes available that may be relevant to the subject's willingness to continue participation in the trial.

(q) The person(s) to contact for further information regarding the trial and the rights of trial subjects, and whom to contact in the event of trial-related injury.

(r) The foreseeable circumstances and/or reasons under which the subject's participation in the trial may be terminated.

(s) The expected duration of the subject's participation in the trial.

(t) The approximate number of subjects involved in the trial.

4.8.11 Prior to participation in the trial, the subject or the subject's legally acceptable representative should receive a copy of the signed and dated written informed consent form and any other written information provided to the subjects. During a subject's participation in the trial, the subject or the subject's legally acceptable representative should receive a copy of the signed and dated consent form updates and a copy of any amendments to the written information provided to subjects.

4.8.12 When a clinical trial (therapeutic or nontherapeutic) includes subjects who can only be enrolled in the trial with the consent of the subject's legally acceptable representative (e.g., minors, or patients with severe dementia), the subject should be informed about the trial to the extent compatible with the subject's understanding and, if capable, the subject should assent, sign and personally date the written informed consent.

4.8.13 Except as described in 4.8.14, a nontherapeutic trial (i.e., a trial in which there is no anticipated direct clinical benefit to the subject) should be conducted in subjects who personally give consent and who sign and date the written informed consent form.

4.8.14 Nontherapeutic trials may be conducted in subjects with consent of a legally acceptable representative provided the following conditions are fulfilled:

(a) The objectives of the trial cannot be met by means of a trial in subjects who can give informed consent personally.

(b) The foreseeable risks to the subjects are low.

(c) The negative impact on the subject's well-being is minimized and low.

(d) The trial is not prohibited by law.

(e) The approval/favorable opinion of the IRB/IEC is expressly sought on the inclusion of such subjects, and the written approval/favorable opinion covers this aspect.

Such trials, unless an exception is justified, should be conducted in patients having a disease or condition for which the investigational product is intended. Subjects in these trials should be particularly closely monitored and should be withdrawn if they appear to be unduly distressed.

4.8.15 In emergency situations, when prior consent of the subject is not possible, the consent of the subject's legally acceptable representative, if present, should be requested. When prior consent of the subject is not possible, and the subject's legally acceptable representative is not available, enrollment of the subject should require measures described in the protocol and/or elsewhere, with documented approval/favorable opinion by the IRB/IEC, to protect the rights, safety, and well-being of the subject and to ensure compliance with applicable regulatory requirements. The subject or the subject's legally acceptable representative should be informed about the trial as soon as possible and consent to continue and other consent as appropriate (see section 4.8.10) should be requested.

4.9 Records and Reports

4.9.1 The investigator should ensure the accuracy, completeness, legibility, and timeliness of the data reported to the sponsor in the CRFs and in all required reports.

4.9.2 Data reported on the CRF, which are derived from source documents, should be consistent with the source documents or the discrepancies should be explained.

4.9.3 Any change or correction to a CRF should be dated, initialed, and explained (if necessary) and should not obscure the original entry (i.e., an audit trail should be maintained); this applies to both written and electronic changes or corrections (see section 5.18.4(n)). Sponsors should provide guidance to investigators and/or the investigators' designated representatives on making such corrections. Sponsors should have written procedures to assure that changes or corrections in CRFs made by sponsor's designated representatives are documented, are necessary, and are endorsed by the investigator. The investigator should retain records of the changes and corrections.

4.9.4 The investigator/institution should maintain the trial documents as specified in Essential Documents for the Conduct of a Clinical Trial (see section 8) and as required by the applicable regulatory requirement(s). The investigator/institution should take measures to prevent accidental or premature destruction of these documents.

4.9.5   Essential documents should be retained until at least 2 years after the last approval of a marketing application in an ICH region and until there are no pending or contemplated marketing applications in an ICH region or at least 2 years have elapsed since the formal discontinuation of clinical development of the investigational product. These documents should be retained for a longer period, however, if required by the applicable regulatory requirements or by an agreement with the sponsor. It is the responsibility of the sponsor to inform the investigator/institution as to when these documents no longer need to be retained (see section 5.5.12).

4.9.6   The financial aspects of the trial should be documented in an agreement between the sponsor and the investigator/institution.

4.9.7   Upon request of the monitor, auditor, IRB/IEC, or regulatory authority, the investigator/institution should make available for direct access all requested trial-related records.

4.10 Progress Reports

4.10.1   Where required by the applicable regulatory requirements, the investigator should submit written summaries of the trial's status to the institution. The investigator/institution should submit written summaries of the status of the trial to the IRB/IEC annually, or more frequently, if requested by the IRB/IEC.

4.10.2   The investigator should promptly provide written reports to the sponsor, the IRB/IEC (see section 3.3.8), and, where required by the applicable regulatory requirements, the institution on any changes significantly affecting the conduct of the trial, and/or increasing the risk to subjects.

4.11 Safety Reporting

4.11.1   All serious adverse events (SAEs) should be reported immediately to the sponsor except for those SAEs that the protocol or other document (e.g., Investigator's Brochure) identifies as not needing immediate reporting. The immediate reports should be followed promptly by detailed, written reports. The immediate and follow-up reports should identify subjects by unique code numbers assigned to the trial subjects rather than by the subjects' names, personal identification numbers, and/or addresses. The investigator should also comply with the applicable regulatory requirement(s) related to the reporting of unexpected serious adverse drug reactions to the regulatory authority(ies) and the IRB/IEC.

4.11.2   Adverse events and/or laboratory abnormalities identified in the protocol as critical to safety evaluations should be reported to the sponsor according to the reporting requirements and within the time periods specified by the sponsor in the protocol.

4.11.3   For reported deaths, the investigator should supply the sponsor and the IRB/IEC with any additional requested information (e.g., autopsy reports and terminal medical reports).

4.12 Premature Termination or Suspension of a Trial

If the trial is terminated prematurely or suspended for any reason, the investigator/institution should promptly inform the trial subjects, should assure appropriate therapy and follow-up for the subjects, and, where required by the applicable regulatory requirement(s), should inform the regulatory authority(ies). In addition:

4.12.1   If the investigator terminates or suspends a trial without prior agreement of the sponsor, the investigator should inform the institution, where required by the applicable regulatory requirements, and the investigator/institution should promptly inform the sponsor and the IRB/IEC, and should provide the sponsor and the IRB/IEC a detailed written explanation of the termination or suspension.

4.12.2   If the sponsor terminates or suspends a trial (see section 5.21), the investigator should promptly inform the institution, where required by the applicable regulatory requirements, and the investigator/institution should promptly inform the IRB/IEC and provide the IRB/IEC a detailed written explanation of the termination or suspension.

4.12.3   If the IRB/IEC terminates or suspends its approval/favorable opinion of a trial (see sections 3.1.2 and 3.3.9), the investigator should inform the institution, where required by the applicable regulatory requirements, and the investigator/institution should promptly notify the sponsor and provide the sponsor with a detailed written explanation of the termination or suspension.

4.13 Final Report(s) by Investigator/Institution

Upon completion of the trial, the investigator should, where required by the applicable regulatory requirements, inform the institution, and the investigator/institution should provide the sponsor with all required reports, the IRB/IEC with a summary of the trial's outcome, and the regulatory authority(ies) with any report(s) they require of the investigator/institution.

5. SPONSOR

5.1 Quality Assurance and Quality Control

5.1.1   The sponsor is responsible for implementing and maintaining quality assurance and quality control systems with written SOPs to ensure that trials are conducted and data are generated, documented (recorded), and reported in compliance with the protocol, GCP, and the applicable regulatory requirement(s).

5.1.2   The sponsor is responsible for securing agreement from all involved parties to ensure direct access (see section 1.21) to all trial-related sites, source data/documents, and reports for the purpose of monitoring and auditing by the sponsor, and inspection by domestic and foreign regulatory authorities.

5.1.3   Quality control should be applied to each stage of data handling to ensure that all data are reliable and have been processed correctly.

5.1.4   Agreements, made by the sponsor with the investigator/institution and/or with any other parties involved with the clinical trial, should be in writing, as part of the protocol or in a separate agreement.

5.2 Contract Research Organization (CRO)

5.2.1   A sponsor may transfer any or all of the sponsor's trial-related duties and functions to a CRO, but the ultimate responsibility for the quality and integrity of the trial data always resides with the sponsor. The CRO should implement quality assurance and quality control.

5.2.2   Any trial-related duty and function that is transferred to and assumed by a CRO should be specified in writing.

5.2.3   Any trial-related duties and functions not specifically transferred to and assumed by a CRO are retained by the sponsor.

5.2.4   All references to a sponsor in this guidance also apply to a CRO to the extent that a CRO has assumed the trial-related duties and functions of a sponsor.

5.3   Medical Expertise

The sponsor should designate appropriately qualified medical personnel who will be readily available to advise on trial-related medical questions or problems. If necessary, outside consultant(s) may be appointed for this purpose.

5.4   Trial Design

5.4.1   The sponsor should utilize qualified individuals (e.g., biostatisticians, clinical pharmacologists, and physicians) as appropriate, throughout all stages of the trial process, from designing the protocol and CRFs and planning the analyses to analyzing and preparing interim and final clinical trial/study reports.

5.4.2   For further guidance: Clinical Trial Protocol and Protocol Amendment(s) (see section 6), the ICH Guidance for Structure and Content of Clinical Study Reports, and other appropriate ICH guidance on trial design, protocol, and conduct.

5.5   Trial Management, Data Handling, Recordkeeping, and Independent Data Monitoring Committee

5.5.1   The sponsor should utilize appropriately qualified individuals to supervise the overall conduct of the trial, to handle the data, to verify the data, to conduct the statistical analyses, and to prepare the trial reports.

5.5.2   The sponsor may consider establishing an independent data monitoring committee (IDMC) to assess the progress of a clinical trial, including the safety data and the critical efficacy endpoints at intervals, and to recommend to the sponsor whether to continue, modify, or stop a trial. The IDMC should have written operating procedures and maintain written records of all its meetings.

5.5.3   When using electronic trial data handling and/or remote electronic trial data systems, the sponsor should:

(a) Ensure and document that the electronic data processing system(s) conforms to the sponsor's established requirements for completeness, accuracy, reliability, and consistent intended performance (i.e., validation).

(b) Maintain SOPs for using these systems.

(c) Ensure that the systems are designed to permit data changes in such a way that the data changes are documented and that there is no deletion of entered data (i.e., maintain an audit trail, data trail, edit trail).

(d) Maintain a security system that prevents unauthorized access to the data.

(e) Maintain a list of the individuals who are authorized to make data changes (see sections 4.1.5 and 4.9.3).

(f) Maintain adequate backup of the data.

(g) Safeguard the blinding, if any (e.g., maintain the blinding during data entry and processing).

5.5.4   If data are transformed during processing, it should always be possible to compare the original data and observations with the processed data.

5.5.5   The sponsor should use an unambiguous subject identification code (see section 1.58) that allows identification of all the data reported for each subject.

5.5.6   The sponsor, or other owners of the data, should retain all of the sponsor- specific essential documents pertaining to the trial. (See section 8. "Essential Documents for the Conduct of a Clinical Trial.")

5.5.7   The sponsor should retain all sponsor-specific essential documents in conformance with the applicable regulatory requirement(s) of the country(ies) where the product is approved, and/or where the sponsor intends to apply for approval(s).

5.5.8   If the sponsor discontinues the clinical development of an investigational product (i.e., for any or all indications, routes of administration, or dosage forms), the sponsor should maintain all sponsor-specific essential documents for at least 2 years after formal discontinuation or in conformance with the applicable regulatory requirement(s).

5.5.9   If the sponsor discontinues the clinical development of an investigational product, the sponsor should notify all the trial investigators/institutions and all the appropriate regulatory authorities.

5.5.10   Any transfer of ownership of the data should be reported to the appropriate authority(ies), as required by the applicable regulatory requirement(s).

5.5.11   The sponsor-specific essential documents should be retained until at least 2 years after the last approval of a marketing application in an ICH region and until there are no pending or contemplated marketing applications in an ICH region or at least 2 years have elapsed since the formal discontinuation of clinical development of the investigational product. These documents should be retained for a longer period, however, if required by the applicable regulatory requirement(s) or if needed by the sponsor.

5.5.12   The sponsor should inform the investigator(s)/institution(s) in writing of the need for record retention and should notify the investigator(s)/ institution(s) in writing when the trial-related records are no longer needed (see section 4.9.5).

5.6   Investigator Selection

5.6.1   The sponsor is responsible for selecting the investigator(s)/ institution(s). Each investigator should be qualified by training and experience and should have adequate resources (see sections 4.1, 4.2) to properly conduct the trial for which the investigator is selected. If a coordinating committee and/or coordinating investigator(s) are to be utilized in multicenter trials, their organization and/or selection are the sponsor's responsibility.

5.6.2 Before entering an agreement with an investigator/institution to conduct a trial, the sponsor should provide the investigator(s)/institution(s) with the protocol and an up-to-date Investigator's Brochure, and should provide sufficient time for the investigator/institution to review the protocol and the information provided.

5.6.3 The sponsor should obtain the investigator's/institution's agreement:

(a) To conduct the trial in compliance with GCP, with the applicable regulatory requirement(s), and with the protocol agreed to by the sponsor and given approval/favorable opinion by the IRB/IEC;

(b) To comply with procedures for data recording/reporting;

(c) To permit monitoring, auditing, and inspection (see section 4.1.4); and

(d) To retain the essential documents that should be in the investigator/institution files (see section 8.) until the sponsor informs the investigator/institution these documents are no longer needed (see sections 4.9.4, 4.9.5, and 5.5.12).

The sponsor and the investigator/institution should sign the protocol, or an alternative document, to confirm this agreement.

5.7 Allocation of Duties and Functions

Prior to initiating a trial, the sponsor should define, establish, and allocate all trial-related duties and functions.

5.8 Compensation to Subjects and Investigators

5.8.1 If required by the applicable regulatory requirement(s), the sponsor should provide insurance or should indemnify (legal and financial coverage) the investigator/institution against claims arising from the trial, except for claims that arise from malpractice and/or negligence.

5.8.2 The sponsor's policies and procedures should address the costs of treatment of trial subjects in the event of trial-related injuries in accordance with the applicable regulatory requirement(s).

5.8.3 When trial subjects receive compensation, the method and manner of compensation should comply with applicable regulatory requirement(s).

5.9 Financing

The financial aspects of the trial should be documented in an agreement between the sponsor and the investigator/institution.

5.10 Notification/Submission to Regulatory Authority(ies)

Before initiating the clinical trial(s), the sponsor (or the sponsor and the investigator, if required by the applicable regulatory requirement(s)), should submit any required application(s) to the appropriate authority(ies) for review, acceptance, and/or permission (as required by the applicable regulatory requirement(s)) to begin the trial(s). Any notification/submission should be dated and contain sufficient information to identify the protocol.

5.11 Confirmation of Review by IRB/IEC

5.11.1 The sponsor should obtain from the investigator/institution:

(a) The name and address of the investigator's/institution's IRB/IEC.

(b) A statement obtained from the IRB/IEC that it is organized and operates according to GCP and the applicable laws and regulations.

(c) Documented IRB/IEC approval/favorable opinion and, if requested by the sponsor, a current copy of protocol, written informed consent form(s) and any other written information to be provided to subjects, subject recruiting procedures, and documents related to payments and compensation available to the subjects, and any other documents that the IRB/IEC may have requested.

5.11.2 If the IRB/IEC conditions its approval/favorable opinion upon change(s) in any aspect of the trial, such as modification(s) of the protocol, written informed consent form and any other written information to be provided to subjects, and/or other procedures, the sponsor should obtain from the investigator/institution a copy of the modification(s) made and the date approval/favorable opinion was given by the IRB/IEC.

5.11.3 The sponsor should obtain from the investigator/institution documentation and dates of any IRB/IEC reapprovals/reevaluations with favorable opinion, and of any withdrawals or suspensions of approval/favorable opinion.

5.12 Information on Investigational Product(s)

5.12.1 When planning trials, the sponsor should ensure that sufficient safety and efficacy data from nonclinical studies and/or clinical trials are available to support human exposure by the route, at the dosages, for the duration, and in the trial population to be studied.

5.12.2 The sponsor should update the Investigator's Brochure as significant new information becomes available. (See section 7. "Investigator's Brochure.")

5.13 Manufacturing, Packaging, Labeling, and Coding Investigational Product(s)

5.13.1 The sponsor should ensure that the investigational product(s) (including active comparator(s) and placebo, if applicable) is characterized as appropriate to the stage of development of the product(s), is manufactured in accordance with any applicable GMP, and is coded and labeled in a manner that protects the blinding, if applicable. In addition, the labeling should comply with applicable regulatory requirement(s).

5.13.2 The sponsor should determine, for the investigational product(s), acceptable storage temperatures, storage conditions (e.g., protection from light), storage times, reconstitution fluids and procedures, and devices for product infusion, if any. The sponsor should inform all involved parties (e.g., monitors, investigators, pharmacists, storage managers) of these determinations.

5.13.3 The investigational product(s) should be packaged to prevent contamination and unacceptable deterioration during transport and storage.

5.13.4 In blinded trials, the coding system for the investigational product(s) should include a mechanism that permits rapid identification of the product(s) in case of a medical emergency, but does not permit undetectable breaks of the blinding.

5.13.5 If significant formulation changes are made in the investigational or comparator product(s) during the course of clinical development, the results of any additional studies of the formulated product(s) (e.g., stability, dissolution rate, bioavailability) needed to assess whether these changes would significantly alter the pharmacokinetic profile of the product should be available prior to the use of the new formulation in clinical trials.

5.14 Supplying and Handling Investigational Product(s)

5.14.1 The sponsor is responsible for supplying the investigator(s)/institution(s) with the investigational product(s).

5.14.2 The sponsor should not supply an investigator/institution with the investigational product(s) until the sponsor obtains all required documentation (e.g., approval/favorable opinion from IRB/IEC and regulatory authority(ies)).

5.14.3 The sponsor should ensure that written procedures include instructions that the investigator/institution should follow for the handling and storage of investigational product(s) for the trial and documentation thereof. The procedures should address adequate and safe receipt, handling, storage, dispensing, retrieval of unused product from subjects, and return of unused investigational product(s) to the sponsor (or alternative disposition if authorized by the sponsor and in compliance with the applicable regulatory requirement(s)).

5.14.4 The sponsor should:

(a) Ensure timely delivery of investigational product(s) to the investigator(s).

(b) Maintain records that document shipment, receipt, disposition, return, and destruction of the investigational product(s). (See section 8. "Essential Documents for the Conduct of a Clinical Trial.")

(c) Maintain a system for retrieving investigational products and documenting this retrieval (e.g., for deficient product recall, reclaim after trial completion, expired product reclaim).

(d) Maintain a system for the disposition of unused investigational product(s) and for the documentation of this disposition.

5.14.5 The sponsor should:

(a) Take steps to ensure that the investigational product(s) is stable over the period of use.

(b) Maintain sufficient quantities of the investigational product(s) used in the trials to reconfirm specifications, should this become necessary, and maintain records of batch sample analyses and characteristics. To the extent stability permits, samples should be retained either until the analyses of the trial data are complete or as required by the applicable regulatory requirement(s), whichever represents the longer retention period.

5.15 Record Access

5.15.1 The sponsor should ensure that it is specified in the protocol or other written agreement that the investigator(s)/institution(s) provide direct access to source data/documents for trial-related monitoring, audits, IRB/IEC review, and regulatory inspection.

5.15.2 The sponsor should verify that each subject has consented, in writing, to direct access to his/her original medical records for trial-related monitoring, audit, IRB/IEC review, and regulatory inspection.

5.16 Safety Information

5.16.1 The sponsor is responsible for the ongoing safety evaluation of the investigational product(s).

5.16.2 The sponsor should promptly notify all concerned investigator(s)/institution(s) and the regulatory authority(ies) of findings that could affect adversely the safety of subjects, impact the conduct of the trial, or alter the IRB/IEC's approval/favorable opinion to continue the trial.

5.17 Adverse Drug Reaction Reporting

5.17.1 The sponsor should expedite the reporting to all concerned investigator(s)/institutions(s), to the IRB(s)/IEC(s), where required, and to the regulatory authority(ies) of all adverse drug reactions (ADRs) that are both serious and unexpected.

5.17.2 Such expedited reports should comply with the applicable regulatory requirement(s) and with the ICH Guidance for Clinical Safety Data Management: Definitions and Standards for Expedited Reporting.

5.17.3 The sponsor should submit to the regulatory authority(ies) all safety updates and periodic reports, as required by applicable regulatory requirement(s).

5.18 Monitoring

5.18.1 **Purpose** The purposes of trial monitoring are to verify that:

(a) The rights and well-being of human subjects are protected.

(b) The reported trial data are accurate, complete, and verifiable from source documents.

(c) The conduct of the trial is in compliance with the currently approved protocol/amendments), with GCP, and with applicable regulatory requirement(s).

5.18.2 **Selection and Qualifications of Monitors**

(a) Monitors should be appointed by the sponsor.

(b) Monitors should be appropriately trained, and should have the scientific and/or clinical knowledge needed to monitor the trial adequately. A monitor's qualifications should be documented.

(c) Monitors should be thoroughly familiar with the investigational product(s), the protocol, written informed consent form and any other written information to be provided to subjects, the sponsor's SOPs, GCP, and the applicable regulatory requirement(s).

5.18.3 **Extent and Nature of Monitoring**

The sponsor should ensure that the trials are adequately monitored. The sponsor should determine the appropriate extent and nature of monitoring. The determination of the extent and nature of monitoring should be based on considerations such as the objective, purpose, design, complexity, blinding, size, and endpoints of the trial. In general there is a need for on-site monitoring, before, during, and after the trial; however, in exceptional circumstances the sponsor may determine that central monitoring in conjunction with procedures such as investigators' training and meetings, and extensive written guidance can assure appropriate conduct of the trial in accordance with GCP. Statistically controlled sampling may be an acceptable method for selecting the data to be verified.

5.18.4 **Monitor's Responsibilities**

The monitor(s), in accordance with the sponsor's requirements, should ensure that the trial is conducted and documented properly by carrying out the following activities when relevant and necessary to the trial and the trial site:

(a)   Acting as the main line of communication between the sponsor and the investigator.

(b)   Verifying that the investigator has adequate qualifications and resources (see sections 4.1, 4.2, 5.6) and these remain adequate throughout the trial period, and that the staff and facilities, including laboratories and equipment, are adequate to safely and properly conduct the trial and these remain adequate throughout the trial period.

(c)   Verifying, for the investigational product(s):

(i)   That storage times and conditions are acceptable, and that supplies are sufficient throughout the trial.

(ii)   That the investigational product(s) is supplied only to subjects who are eligible to receive it and at the protocol specified dose(s).

(iii)   That subjects are provided with necessary instruction on properly using, handling, storing, and returning the investigational product(s).

(iv)   That the receipt, use, and return of the investigational product(s) at the trial sites are controlled and documented adequately.

(v)   That the disposition of unused investigational product(s) at the trial sites complies with applicable regulatory requirement(s) and is in accordance with the sponsor's authorized procedures.

(d)   Verifying that the investigator follows the approved protocol and all approved amendment(s), if any.

(e)   Verifying that written informed consent was obtained before each subject's participation in the trial.

(f)   Ensuring that the investigator receives the current Investigator's Brochure, all documents, and all trial supplies needed to conduct the trial properly and to comply with the applicable regulatory requirement(s).

(g)   Ensuring that the investigator and the investigator's trial staff are adequately informed about the trial.

(h)   Verifying that the investigator and the investigator's trial staff are performing the specified trial functions, in accordance with the protocol and any other written agreement between the sponsor and the investigator/institution, and have not delegated these functions to unauthorized individuals.

(i)   Verifying that the investigator is enrolling only eligible subjects.

(j)   Reporting the subject recruitment rate.

(k)   Verifying that source data/documents and other trial records are accurate, complete, kept up-to-date, and maintained.

(l)   Verifying that the investigator provides all the required reports, notifications, applications, and submissions, and that these documents are accurate, complete, timely, legible, dated, and identify the trial.

(m) Checking the accuracy and completeness of the CRF entries, source data/documents, and other trial-related records against each other. The monitor specifically should verify that:

(i)   The data required by the protocol are reported accurately on the CRFs and are consistent with the source data/documents.

(ii)   Any dose and/or therapy modifications are well documented for each of the trial subjects.

(iii) Adverse events, concomitant medications, and intercurrent illnesses are reported in accordance with the protocol on the CRFs.

(iv) Visits that the subjects fail to make, tests that are not conducted, and examinations that are not performed are clearly reported as such on the CRFs.

(v)   All withdrawals and dropouts of enrolled subjects from the trial are reported and explained on the CRFs.

(n)   Informing the investigator of any CRF entry error, omission, or illegibility. The monitor should ensure that appropriate corrections, additions, or deletions are made, dated, explained (if necessary), and initialed by the investigator or by a member of the investigator's trial staff who is authorized to initial CRF changes for the investigator. This authorization should be documented.

(o)   Determining whether all adverse events (AEs) are appropriately reported within the time periods required by GCP, the ICH Guidance for Clinical Safety Data Management: Definitions and Standards for Expedited Reporting, the protocol, the IRB/IEC, the sponsor, and the applicable regulatory requirement(s).

(p)   Determining whether the investigator is maintaining the essential documents. (See section 8. "Essential Documents for the Conduct of a Clinical Trial.")

(q)   Communicating deviations from the protocol, SOPs, GCP, and the applicable regulatory requirements to the investigator and taking appropriate action designed to prevent recurrence of the detected deviations.

5.18.5 Monitoring Procedures

The monitor(s) should follow the sponsor's established written SOPs as well as those procedures that are specified by the sponsor for monitoring a specific trial.

5.18.6 Monitoring Report

(a) The monitor should submit a written report to the sponsor after each trial-site visit or trial-related communication.

(b) Reports should include the date, site, name of the monitor, and name of the investigator or other individual(s) contacted.

(c) Reports should include a summary of what the monitor reviewed and the monitor's statements concerning the significant findings/facts, deviations and deficiencies, conclusions, actions taken or to be taken, and/or actions recommended to secure compliance.

(d) The review and follow-up of the monitoring report by the sponsor should be documented by the sponsor's designated representative.

5.19 Audit

If or when sponsors perform audits, as part of implementing quality assurance, they should consider:

5.19.1 Purpose

The purpose of a sponsor's audit, which is independent of and separate from routine monitoring or quality control functions, should be to evaluate trial conduct and compliance with the protocol, SOPs, GCP, and the applicable regulatory requirements.

5.19.2 Selection and Qualification of Auditors

(a) The sponsor should appoint individuals, who are independent of the clinical trial/data collection system(s), to conduct audits.

(b) The sponsor should ensure that the auditors are qualified by training and experience to conduct audits properly. An auditor's qualifications should be documented.

5.19.3 Auditing Procedures

(a) The sponsor should ensure that the auditing of clinical trials/ systems is conducted in accordance with the sponsor's written procedures on what to audit, how to audit, the frequency of audits, and the form and content of audit reports.

(b) The sponsor's audit plan and procedures for a trial audit should be guided by the importance of the trial to submissions to regulatory authorities, the number of subjects in the trial, the type and complexity of the trial, the level of risks to the trial subjects, and any identified problem(s).

(c) The observations and findings of the auditor(s) should be documented.

(d) To preserve the independence and value of the audit function, the regulatory authority(ies) should not routinely request the audit reports. Regulatory authority(ies) may seek access to an audit report on a case-by-case basis, when evidence of serious GCP noncompliance exists, or in the course of legal proceedings.

(e) Where required by applicable law or regulation, the sponsor should provide an audit certificate.

5.20 Noncompliance

5.20.1 Noncompliance with the protocol, SOPs, GCP, and/or applicable regulatory requirement(s) by an investigator/institution, or by member(s) of the sponsor's staff should lead to prompt action by the sponsor to secure compliance.

5.20.2 If the monitoring and/or auditing identifies serious and/or persistent noncompliance on the part of an investigator/institution, the sponsor should terminate the investigator's/institution's participation in the trial. When an investigator's/institution's participation is terminated because of noncompliance, the sponsor should notify promptly the regulatory authority(ies).

5.21 Premature Termination or Suspension of a Trial

If a trial is terminated prematurely or suspended, the sponsor should promptly inform the investigators/institutions, and the regulatory authority(ies) of the termination or suspension and the reason(s) for the termination or suspension. The IRB/IEC should also be informed promptly and provide the reason(s) for the termination or suspension by the sponsor or by the investigator/institution, as specified by the applicable regulatory requirement(s).

5.22 Clinical Trial/Study Reports

Whether the trial is completed or prematurely terminated, the sponsor should ensure that the clinical trial/study reports are prepared and provided to the regulatory agency(ies) as required by the applicable regulatory requirement(s). The sponsor should also ensure that the clinical trial/study reports in marketing applications meet the standards of the ICH Guidance for Structure and Content of Clinical Study Reports. (NOTE: The ICH Guidance for Structure and Content of Clinical Study Reports specifies that abbreviated study reports may be acceptable in certain cases.)

5.23 Multicenter Trials

For multicenter trials, the sponsor should ensure that:

5.23.1   All investigators conduct the trial in strict compliance with the protocol agreed to by the sponsor and, if required, by the regulatory authority(ies), and given approval/favorable opinion by the IRB/IEC.

5.23.2   The CRFs are designed to capture the required data at all multicenter trial sites. For those investigators who are collecting additional data, supplemental CRFs should also be provided that are designed to capture the additional data.

5.23.3   The responsibilities of the coordinating investigator(s) and the other participating investigators are documented prior to the start of the trial.

5.23.4   All investigators are given instructions on following the protocol, on complying with a uniform set of standards for the assessment of clinical and laboratory findings, and on completing the CRFs.

5.23.5   Communication between investigators is facilitated.

6. CLINICAL TRIAL PROTOCOL AND PROTOCOL

The contents of a trial protocol should generally include the following topics. However, site specific information may be provided on separate protocol page(s), or addressed in a separate agreement, and some of the information listed below may be contained in other protocol referenced documents, such as an Investigator's Brochure.

6.1 General Information

6.1.1   Protocol title, protocol identifying number, and date. Any amendment(s) should also bear the amendment number(s) and date(s).

6.1.2   Name and address of the sponsor and monitor (if other than the sponsor).

6.1.3   Name and title of the person(s) authorized to sign the protocol and the protocol amendment(s) for the sponsor.

6.1.4   Name, title, address, and telephone number(s) of the sponsor's medical expert (or dentist when appropriate) for the trial.

6.1.5   Name and title of the investigator(s) who is (are) responsible for conducting the trial, and the address and telephone number(s) of the trial site(s).

6.1.6   Name, title, address, and telephone number(s) of the qualified physician (or dentist, if applicable) who is responsible for all trial-site related medical (or dental) decisions (if other than investigator).

6.1.7   Name(s) and address(es) of the clinical laboratory(ies) and other medical and/or technical department(s) and/or institutions involved in the trial.

6.2   Background Information

6.2.1   Name and description of the investigational product(s).

6.2.2   A summary of findings from nonclinical studies that potentially have clinical significance and from clinical trials that are relevant to the trial.

6.2.3   Summary of the known and potential risks and benefits, if any, to human subjects.

6.2.4   Description of and justification for the route of administration, dosage, dosage regimen, and treatment period(s).

6.2.5   A statement that the trial will be conducted in compliance with the protocol, GCP, and the applicable regulatory requirement(s).

6.2.6   Description of the population to be studied.

6.2.7   References to literature and data that are relevant to the trial, and that provide background for the trial.

6.3   Trial Objectives and Purpose

A detailed description of the objectives and the purpose of the trial.

6.4   Trial Design

The scientific integrity of the trial and the credibility of the data from the trial depend substantially on the trial design. A description of the trial design should include:

6.4.1   A specific statement of the primary endpoints and the secondary end-points, if any, to be measured during the trial.

6.4.2   A description of the type/design of trial to be conducted (e.g., double-blind, placebo-controlled, parallel design) and a schematic diagram of trial design, procedures, and stages.

6.4.3   A description of the measures taken to minimize/avoid bias, including (for example):

(a) Randomization.

(b) Blinding.

6.4.4   A description of the trial treatment(s) and the dosage and dosage regimen of the investigational product(s). Also include a description of the dosage form, packaging, and labeling of the investigational product(s).

6.4.5   The expected duration of subject participation, and a description of the sequence and duration of all trial periods, including follow-up, if any.

6.4.6   A description of the "stopping rules" or "discontinuation criteria" for individual subjects, parts of trial, and entire trial.

6.4.7   Accountability procedures for the investigational product(s), including the placebo(s) and comparator(s), if any.

6.4.8   Maintenance of trial treatment randomization codes and procedures for breaking codes.

6.4.9 The identification of any data to be recorded directly on the CRFs (i.e., no prior written or electronic record of data), and to be considered to be source data.

6.5 Selection and Withdrawal of Subjects

6.5.1 Subject inclusion criteria.

6.5.2 Subject exclusion criteria.

6.5.3 Subject withdrawal criteria (i.e., terminating investigational product treatment/trial treatment) and procedures specifying:

(a) When and how to withdraw subjects from the trial/ investigational product treatment.

(b) The type and timing of the data to be collected for withdrawn subjects.

(c) Whether and how subjects are to be replaced.

(d) The follow-up for subjects withdrawn from investigational product treatment/trial treatment.

6.6 Treatment of Subjects

6.6.1 The treatment(s) to be administered, including the name(s) of all the product(s), the dose(s), the dosing schedule(s), the route/mode(s) of administration, and the treatment period(s), including the follow-up period(s) for subjects for each investigational product treatment/trial treatment group/arm of the trial.

6.6.2 Medication(s)/treatment(s) permitted (including rescue medication) and not permitted before and/or during the trial.

6.6.3 Procedures for monitoring subject compliance.

6.7 Assessment of Efficacy

6.7.1 Specification of the efficacy parameters.

6.7.2 Methods and timing for assessing, recording, and analyzing efficacy parameters.

6.8 Assessment of Safety

6.8.1 Specification of safety parameters.

6.8.2 The methods and timing for assessing, recording, and analyzing safety parameters.

6.8.3 Procedures for eliciting reports of and for recording and reporting adverse event and intercurrent illnesses.

6.8.4 The type and duration of the follow-up of subjects after adverse events.

6.9 Statistics

6.9.1 A description of the statistical methods to be employed, including timing of any planned interim analysis(ses).

6.9.2 The number of subjects planned to be enrolled. In multicenter trials, the number of enrolled subjects projected for each trial site should be specified. Reason for choice of sample size, including reflections on (or calculations of) the power of the trial and clinical justification.

6.9.3 The level of significance to be used.

6.9.4   Criteria for the termination of the trial.

6.9.5   Procedure for accounting for missing, unused, and spurious data.

6.9.6   Procedures for reporting any deviation(s) from the original statistical plan (any deviation(s) from the original statistical plan should be described and justified in the protocol and/or in the final report, as appropriate).

6.9.7   The selection of subjects to be included in the analyses (e.g., all randomized subjects, all dosed subjects, all eligible subjects, evaluate-able subjects).

6.10 Direct Access to Source Data/Documents

The sponsor should ensure that it is specified in the protocol or other written agreement that the investigator(s)/institution(s) will permit trial-related monitoring, audits, IRB/IEC review, and regulatory inspection(s) by providing direct access to source data/documents.

6.11 Quality Control and Quality Assurance

6.12 Ethics

Description of ethical considerations relating to the trial.

6.13 Data Handling and Recordkeeping

6.14 Financing and Insurance

Financing and insurance if not addressed in a separate agreement.

6.15 Publication Policy

Publication policy, if not addressed in a separate agreement.

6.16 Supplements

(NOTE: Since the protocol and the clinical trial/study report are closely related, further relevant information can be found in the ICH Guidance for Structure and Content of Clinical Study Reports.)

7. INVESTIGATOR'S BROCHURE

7.1 Introduction

The Investigator's Brochure (IB) is a compilation of the clinical and nonclinical data on the investigational product(s) that are relevant to the study of the product(s) in human subjects. Its purpose is to provide the investigators and others involved in the trial with the information to facilitate their understanding of the rationale for, and their compliance with, many key features of the protocol, such as the dose, dose frequency/interval, methods of administration, and safety monitoring procedures. The IB also provides insight to support the clinical management of the study subjects during the course of the clinical trial. The information should be presented in a concise, simple, objective, balanced, and nonpromotional form that enables a clinician, or potential investigator, to understand it and make his/her own unbiased risk-benefit assessment of the appropriateness of the proposed trial. For this reason, a medically qualified person should generally participate in the editing of an IB, but the contents of the IB should be approved by the disciplines that generated the described data.

This guidance delineates the minimum information that should be included in an IB and provides suggestions for its layout. It is expected that the type and extent of information available will vary with the stage of development of the investigational product. If the investigational product is marketed and its pharmacology is widely understood by medical practitioners, an extensive IB may not be necessary. Where permitted by regulatory authorities, a basic product information brochure, package leaflet, or labeling may be an appropriate alternative, provided that it includes current, comprehensive, and detailed information on all aspects of the investigational product that might be of importance to the investigator. If a marketed product is being studied for a new use (i.e., a new indication), an IB specific to that new use should be prepared. The IB should be reviewed at least annually and revised as necessary in compliance with a sponsor's written procedures. More frequent revision may be appropriate depending on the stage of development and the generation of relevant new information. However, in accordance with GCP, relevant new information may be so important that it should be communicated to the investigators, and possibly to the Institutional Review Boards (IRBs)/Independent Ethics Committees (IECs) and/or regulatory authorities before it is included in a revised IB.

Generally, the sponsor is responsible for ensuring that an up-to-date IB is made available to the investigator(s) and the investigators are responsible for providing the up-to-date IB to the responsible IRBs/IECs. In the case of an investigator-sponsored trial, the sponsor-investigator should determine whether a brochure is available from the commercial manufacturer. If the investigational product is provided by the sponsor-investigator, then he or she should provide the necessary information to the trial personnel. In cases where preparation of a formal IB is impractical, the sponsor-investigator should provide, as a substitute, an expanded background information section in the trial protocol that contains the minimum current information described in this guidance.

7.2 General Considerations

The IB should include:

7.2.1 **Title Page** This should provide the sponsor's name, the identity of each investigational product (i.e., research number, chemical or approved generic name, and trade name(s) where legally permissible and desired by the sponsor), and the release date. It is also suggested that an edition number, and a reference to the number and date of the edition it supersedes, be provided. An example is given in Appendix 1.

7.2.2 **Confidentiality Statement** The sponsor may wish to include a statement instructing the investigator/recipients to treat the IB as a confidential document for the sole information and use of the investigator's team and the IRB/IEC.

7.3 Contents of the Investigator's Brochure

The IB should contain the following sections, each with literature references where appropriate:

7.3.1 **Table of Contents** An example of the Table of Contents is given in Appendix 2.

7.3.2 **Summary** A brief summary (preferably not exceeding two pages) should be given, highlighting the significant physical, chemical, pharmaceutical, pharmacological, lexicological, pharmacokinetic, metabolic, and clinical information available that is relevant to the stage of clinical development of the investigational product.

7.3.3 **Introduction** A brief introductory statement should be provided that contains the chemical name (and generic and trade name(s) when approved) of the investigational product(s), all active ingredients, the investigational product(s) pharmacological class and its expected position within this class (e.g., advantages), the rationale for performing research with the investigational product(s), and the anticipated prophylactic, therapeutic, or diagnostic indication(s). Finally, the introductory statement should provide the general approach to be followed in evaluating the investigational product.

7.3.4 Physical, Chemical, and Pharmaceutical Properties and Formulation

A description should be provided of the investigational product substance(s) (including the chemical and/or structural formula(e)), and a brief summary should be given of the relevant physical, chemical, and pharmaceutical properties.

To permit appropriate safety measures to be taken in the course of the trial, a description of the formulation(s) to be used, including excipients, should be provided and justified if clinically relevant. Instructions for the storage and handling of the dosage form(s) should also be given.

Any structural similarities to other known compounds should be mentioned.

7.3.5 Nonclinical Studies

Introduction:

The results of all relevant nonclinical pharmacology, toxicology, pharmacokinetic, and investigational product metabolism studies should be provided in summary form. This summary should address the methodology used, the results, and a discussion of the relevance of the findings to the investigated therapeutic and the possible unfavorable and unintended effects in humans.

The information provided may include the following, as appropriate, if known/available:

> Species tested;
>
> Number and sex of animals in each group;
>
> Unit dose (e.g., milligram/kilogram (mg/kg));
>
> Dose interval;
>
> Route of administration;
>
> Duration of dosing;
>
> Information on systemic distribution;
>
> Duration of post-exposure follow-up;
>
> Results, including the following aspects:
>
> > - Nature and frequency of pharmacological or toxic effects;
> >
> > - Severity or intensity of pharmacological or toxic effects;
> >
> > - Time to onset of effects;
> >
> > - Reversibility of effects;
> >
> > - Duration of effects;
> >
> > - Dose response.

Tabular format/listings should be used whenever possible to enhance the clarity of the presentation.

The following sections should discuss the most important findings from the studies, including the dose response of observed effects, the relevance to humans, and any aspects to be studied in humans. If applicable, the effective and nontoxic dose findings in the same animal species should be compared (i.e., the therapeutic index should be discussed). The relevance of this information to the proposed human dosing should be addressed. Whenever possible, comparisons should be made in terms of blood/tissue levels rather than on a mg/kg basis.

(a) Nonclinical Pharmacology

A summary of the pharmacological aspects of the investigational product and, where appropriate, its significant metabolites studied in animals should be included. Such a summary should incorporate studies that assess potential therapeutic activity (e.g., efficacy models, receptor binding, and specificity) as well as those that assess safety (e.g., special studies to assess pharmacological actions other than the intended therapeutic effect(s)).

(b) Pharmacokinetics and Product Metabolism in Animals

A summary of the pharmacokinetics and biological transformation and disposition of the investigational product in all species studied should be given. The discussion of the findings should address the absorption and the local and systemic bioavailability of the investigational product and its metabolites, and their relationship to the pharmacological and lexicological findings in animal species.

(c) Toxicology

A summary of the toxicological effects found in relevant studies conducted in different animal species should be described under the following headings where appropriate:

Single dose;

Repeated dose;

Carcinogenicity;

Special studies (e.g., irritancy and sensitization);

Reproductive toxicity;

Genotoxicity (mutagenicity).

7.3.6 **Effects in Humans**

Introduction:

A thorough discussion of the known effects of the investigational product(s) in humans should be provided, including information on pharmacokinetics, metabolism, pharmacodynamics, dose response, safety, efficacy, and other pharmacological activities. Where possible, a summary of each completed clinical trial should be provided. Information should also be provided regarding results from any use of the investigational product(s) other than in clinical trials, such as from experience during marketing.

(a) Pharmacokinetics and Product Metabolism in Humans

A summary of information on the pharmacokinetics of the investigational product(s) should be presented, including the following, if available:

Pharmacokinetics (including metabolism, as appropriate, and absorption, plasma protein binding, distribution, and elimination).

Bioavailability of the investigational product (absolute, where possible, and/or relative) using a reference dosage form.

Population subgroups (e.g., gender, age, and impaired organ function).

Interactions (e.g., product-product interactions and effects of food).

Other pharmacokinetic data (e.g., results of population studies performed within clinical trial(s)).

(b) Safety and Efficacy

A summary of information should be provided about the investigational product's/products' (including metabolites, where appropriate) safety, pharmacodynamics, efficacy, and dose response that were obtained from preceding trials in humans (healthy volunteers and/or patients). The implications of this information should be discussed. In cases where a number of clinical trials have been completed, the use of summaries of safety and efficacy across multiple trials by indications in subgroups may provide a clear presentation of the data. Tabular summaries of adverse drug reactions for all the clinical trials (including those for all the studied indications) would be useful. Important differences in adverse drug reaction patterns/incidences across indications or subgroups should be discussed.

The IB should provide a description of the possible risks and adverse drug reactions to be anticipated on the basis of prior experiences with the product under investigation and with related products. A description should also be provided of the precautions or special monitoring to be done as part of the investigational use of the product(s).

(c) Marketing Experience

The IB should identify countries where the investigational product has been marketed or approved. Any significant information arising from the marketed use should be summarized (e.g., formulations, dosages, routes of administration, and adverse product reactions). The IB should also identify all the countries where the investigational product did not receive approval/registration for marketing or was withdrawn from marketing/registration.

7.3.7 Summary of Data and Guidance for the Investigator

This section should provide an overall discussion of the nonclinical and clinical data, and should summarize the information from various sources on different aspects of the investigational product(s), wherever possible. In this way, the investigator can be provided with the most informative interpretation of the available data and with an assessment of the implications of the information for future clinical trials.

Where appropriate, the published reports on related products should be discussed. This could help the investigator to anticipate adverse drug reactions or other problems in clinical trials.

The overall aim of this section is to provide the investigator with a clear understanding of the possible risks and adverse reactions, and of the specific tests, observations, and precautions that may be needed for a clinical trial. This understanding should be based on the available physical, chemical, pharmaceutical, pharmacological, lexicological, and clinical information on the investigational product(s). Guidance should also be provided to the clinical investigator on the recognition and treatment of possible overdose and adverse drug reactions that is based on previous human experience and on the pharmacology of the investigational product.

7.4 Appendix 1

TITLE PAGE OF INVESTIGATOR'S BROCHURE (Example)

Sponsor's Name:

Product:

Research Number:

Name(s): Chemical, Generic (if approved)
Trade Name(s) (if legally permissible and desired by the sponsor)

Edition Number:

Release Date:

Replaces Previous Edition Number:

Date:

7.5 Appendix 2

TABLE OF CONTENTS OF INVESTIGATOR'S BROCHURE (Example)

– Confidentiality Statement (optional)
– Signature Page (optional)

1. Table of Contents
2. Summary
3. Introduction
4. Physical, Chemical, and Pharmaceutical Properties and Formulation
5. Nonclinical Studies

    5.1 Nonclinical Pharmacology
    5.2 Pharmacokinetics and Product Metabolism in Animals
    5.3 Toxicology

6. Effects in Humans

    6.1 Pharmacokinetics and Product Metabolism in Humans
    6.2 Safety and Efficacy
    6.3 Marketing Experience

7. Summary of Data and Guidance for the Investigator

NB: References on   1. Publications
2. Reports
These references should be found at the end of each chapter.
Appendices (if any)

8. ESSENTIAL DOCUMENTS FOR THE CONDUCT OF A CLINICAL TRIAL

8.1 Introduction

Essential Documents are those documents that individually and collectively permit evaluation of the conduct of a trial and the quality of the data produced. These documents serve to demonstrate the compliance of the investigator, sponsor, and monitor with the standards of GCP and with all applicable regulatory requirements.

Essential Documents also serve a number of other important purposes. Filing essential documents at the investigator/institution and sponsor sites in a timely manner can greatly assist in the successful management of a trial by the investigator, sponsor, and monitor. These documents are also the ones that are usually audited by the sponsor's independent audit function and inspected by the regulatory authority(ies) as part of the process to confirm the validity of the trial conduct and the integrity of data collected.

The minimum list of essential documents that has been developed follows. The various documents are grouped in three sections according to the stage of the trial during which they will normally be generated (1) before the clinical phase of the trial commences, (2) during the clinical conduct of the trial, and (3) after completion or termination of the trial. A description is given of the purpose of each document, and whether it should be filed in either the investigator/institution or sponsor files, or both. It is acceptable to combine some of the documents, provided the individual elements are readily identifiable.

Trial master files should be established at the beginning of the trial, both at the investigator/institution's site and at the sponsor's office. A final close-out of a trial can only be done when the monitor has reviewed both investigator/institution and sponsor files and confirmed that all necessary documents are in the appropriate files.

Any or all of the documents addressed in this guidance may be subject to, and should be available for, audit by the sponsor's auditor and inspection by the regulatory authority (ies).

8.2 Before the Clinical Phase of the Trial Commences
During this planning stage the following documents should be generated and should be on file before the trial formally starts.

| | | | Located in Files of | |
| | | | Investigator/ Sponsor | Institution |
	Title of Document	Purpose		
8.2.1	Investigator's brochure	To document that relevant and current scientific information about the investigational product has been provided to the investigator	X	X
8.2.2	Signed protocol and amendments, if any, and sample case report form (CRF)	To document investigator and sponsor agreement to the protocol/amendments) and CRF	X	X
8.2.3	Information given to trial subject – Informed consent form (including all applicable translations)	To document the informed consent	X	X
	– Any other written information	To document that subjects will be given appropriate written information (content and wording) to support their ability to give fully informed consent	X	X
	– Advertisement for subject recruitment (if used)	To document that recruitment measures are appropriate and not coercive	X	

	Title of Document	Purpose	Located in Files of	
			Investigator/ Sponsor	Institution
8.2.4	Financial aspects of the trial	To document the financial agreement between the investigator/institution and the sponsor for the trial	X	X
8.2.5	Insurance statement (where required)	To document that compensation to subject(s) for trial-related injury will be available	X	X
8.2.6	Signed agreement between involved parties, e.g.:	To document agreements		
	– Investigator/institution and sponsor		X	X
	– Investigator/institution and CRO		X	X (where required)
	– Sponsor and CRO			X
	– Investigator/institution and authority(ies) (where required)		X	X
8.2.7	Dated, documented approval/favorable opinion of IRB/IEC of the following:	To document that the trial has been subject to IRB/IEC review and given approval/favorable opinion. To identify the version number and date of the document(s).	X	X
	– Protocol and any amendments – CRF (if applicable) – Informed consent form(s) – Any other written information to be provided to the subject(s) – Advertisement for subject recruitment (if used) – Subject compensation (if any) – Any other documents given approval/favorable opinion			
8.2.8	Institutional review board/independent ethics committee composition	To document that the IRB/IEC is constituted in agreement with GCP	X	X (where required)
8.2.9	Regulatory authority(ies) authorization/approval/ notification of protocol (where required)	To document appropriate authorization/approval/ notification by the regulatory authority(ies) has been obtained prior to initiation of the trial in compliance with the applicable regulatory requirement(s)	X (where required)	X (where required)
8.2.10	Curriculum vitae and/or other relevant documents evidencing qualifications of investigator(s) and subinvestigators	To document qualifications and eligibility to conduct trial and/or provide medical supervision of subjects	X	X
8.2.11	Normal value(s)/range(s) for medical/laboratory/technical procedure(s) and/or test(s) included in the protocol	To document normal values and/or ranges of the tests	X	X

	Title of Document	Purpose	Located in Files of	
			Investigator/ Sponsor	Institution
8.2.12	Medical/laboratory/technical procedures/tests – Certification or – Accreditation or – Established quality control and/or external quality assessment or – Other validation (where required)	To document competence of facility to perform required test(s), and support reliability of results	X (where required)	X
8.2.13	Sample of label(s) attached to investigational product container(s)	To document compliance with applicable labeling regulations and appropriateness of instructions provided to the subjects		X
8.2.14	Instructions for handling of investigational product(s) and trial-related materials (if not included in protocol or Investigator' s Brochure)	To document instructions needed to ensure proper storage, packaging, dispensing, and disposition of investigational products and trial-related materials	X	X
8.2.15	Shipping records for investigational product(s) and trial-related materials	To document shipment dates, batch numbers, and method of shipment of investigational product(s) and trial-related materials. Allows tracking of product batch, review of shipping conditions, and accountability.	X	X
8.2.16	Certificate(s) of analysis of investigational product(s) shipped	To document identity, purity, and strength of investigational products to be used in the trial		X
8.2.17	Decoding procedures for blinded trials	To document how, in case of an emergency, identity of blinded investigational product can be revealed without breaking the blind for the remaining subjects' treatment	X	X (third party if applicable)
8.2.18	Master randomization list	To document method for randomization of trial population		X (third party if applicable)
8.2.19	Pretrial monitoring report	To document that the site is suitable for the trial (may be combined with 8.2.20)		X
8.2.20	Trial initiation monitoring report	To document that trial procedures were reviewed with the investigator and investigator's trial staff (may be combined with 8.2.19)	X	X

8.3 During the Clinical Conduct of the Trial

In addition to having on file the above documents, the following should be added to the files during the trial as evidence that all new relevant information is documented as it becomes available.

	Title of Document	Purpose	Located in Files of Investigator/ Sponsor	Institution
8.3.1	Investigator's Brochure updates	To document that investigator is informed in a timely manner of relevant information as it becomes available	X	X
8.3.2	Any revisions to: – Protocol/amendments) and CRF – Informed consent form – Any other written information provided to subjects – Advertisement for subject recruitment (if used)	To document revisions of these trial-related documents that take effect during trial	X	X
8.3.3	Dated, documented approval/favorable opinion of institutional review board (IRB)/independent ethics committee (IEC) of the following: – Protocol amendment(s) – Revision(s) of: – Informed consent form – Any other written information to be provided to the subject – Advertisement for subject recruitment (if used) -Any other documents given approval/favorable opinion – Continuing review of trial (see section 3.1.4)	To document that the amendment(s) and/or revision(s) have been subject to IRB/IEC review and were given approval/favorable opinion. To identify the version number and date of the document(s)	X	X
8.3.4	Regulatory authority(ies) authorizations/ approvals/notifications where required for: – Protocol amendment(s) and other documents	To document compliance with applicable regulatory requirements	X (where required)	X
8.3.5	Curriculum vitae for new investigator(s) and/or subinvestigators	(See section 8.2.10)	X	X

	Title of Document	Purpose	Located in Files of	
			Investigator/ Sponsor	Institution
8.3.6	Updates to normal value(s)/range(s) for medical laboratory /technical procedure(s)/test(s) included in the protocol	To document normal values and ranges that are revised during the trial (see section 8.2.11)	X	X
8.3.7	Updates of medical/ laboratory /technical procedures/tests – Certification or – Accreditation or – Established quality control and/or external quality assessment or – Other validation (where required)	To document that tests remain adequate throughout the trial period (see section 8.2.12)	X (where required)	X
8.3.8	Documentation of investigational product(s) and trial-related materials shipment	(See section 8.2.15)	X	X
8.3.9	Certificate(s) of analysis for new batches of investigational products	(See section 8.2.16)		X
8.3.10	Monitoring visit reports	To document site visits by, and findings of, the monitor		X
8.3.11	Relevant communications other than site visits – Letters – Meeting notes – Notes of telephone calls	To document any agreements or significant discussions regarding trial administration, protocol violations, trial conduct, adverse event (AE) reporting	X	X
8.3.12	Signed informed consent forms	To document that consent is obtained in accordance with GCP and protocol and dated prior to participation of each subject in trial. Also to document direct access permission (see section 8.2.3)	X	
8.3.13	Source documents	To document the existence of the subject and substantiate integrity of trial data collected. To include original documents related to the trial, to medical treatment, and history of subject	X	
8.3.14	Signed, dated, and completed case report forms (CRFs)	To document that the investigator or authorized member of the investigator's staff confirms the observations recorded	X (copy)	X (original)
8.3.15	Documentation of CRF corrections	To document all changes/ additions or corrections made to CRF after initial data were recorded	X (copy)	X (original)

			Located in Files of	
	Title of Document	Purpose	Investigator/ Sponsor	Institution
8.3.16	Notification by originating investigator to sponsor of serious adverse events and related reports	Notification by originating investigator to sponsor of serious adverse events and related reports in accordance with 4.1 1	X	X
8.3.17	Notification by sponsor and/or investigator, where applicable, to regulatory authority(ies) and IRB(s)/IEC(s) of unexpected serious adverse drug reactions and of other safety information	Notification by sponsor and/or investigator, where applicable, to regulatory authorities and IRB(s)/IEC(s) of unexpected serious adverse drug reactions in accordance with 5.17 and 4.11.1 and of other safety information in accordance with 4.11.2 and 5.16.2	X (where required)	X
8.3.18	Notification by sponsor to investigators of safety information	Notification by sponsor to investigators of safety information in accordance with 5.16.2	X	X
8.3.19	Interim or annual reports to IRB/IEC and authority(ies)	Interim or annual reports provided to IRB/IEC in accordance with 4.10 and to authority(ies) in accordance with 5.17.3	X	X (where required)
8.3.20	Subject screening log	To document identification of subjects who entered pretrial screening	X	X (where required)
8.3.21	Subject identification code list	To document that investigator/institution keeps a confidential list of names of all subjects allocated to trial numbers on enrolling in the trial. Allows investigator/ institution to reveal identity of any subject	X	
8.3.22	Subject enrollment log	To document chronological enrollment of subjects by trial number	X	
8.3.23	Investigational product(s) accountability at the site	To document that investigational products(s) have been used according to the protocol	X	X
8.3.24	Signature sheet	To document signatures and initials of all persons authorized to make entries and/or corrections on CRFs	X	X
8.3.25	Record of retained body fluids/tissue samples (if any)	To document location and identification of retained samples if assays need to be repeated	X	X

8.4 After Completion or Termination of the Trial

After completion or termination of the trial, all of the documents identified in sections 8.2 and 8.3 should be in the file together with the following:

	Title of Document	Purpose	Located in Files of Investigator/ Sponsor	Institution
8.4.1	Investigational product(s) accountability at site	To document that the investigational product(s) has been used according to the protocol. To document the final accounting of investigational product(s) received at the site, dispensed to subjects, returned by the subjects, and returned to sponsor	X	X
8.4.2	Documentation of investigational product(s) destruction	To document destruction of unused investigational product(s) by sponsor or at site	X (if destroyed at site)	X
8.4.3	Completed subject identification code list	To permit identification of all subjects enrolled in the trial in case follow-up is required. List should be kept in a confidential manner and for agreed upon time	X	
8.4.4	Audit certificate (if required)	To document that audit was performed (if required) (see section 5.19.3(e))		X
8.4.5	Final trial close-out monitoring report	To document that all activities required for trial close-out are completed, and copies of essential documents are held in the appropriate files		X
8.4.6	Treatment allocation and decoding documentation	Returned to sponsor to document any decoding that may have occurred		X
8.4.7	Final report by investigator/institution to IRB/IEC where required, and where applicable, to the regulatory authority(ies) (see section 4.13)	To document completion of the trial	X	
8.4.8	Clinical study report (see section 5.22)	To document results and interpretation of trial	X (if applicable)	X

WORLD MEDICAL ASSOCIATION DECLARATION OF HELSINKI: ETHICAL PRINCIPLES FOR MEDICAL RESEARCH INVOLVING HUMAN SUBJECTS

Adopted by the 18th WMA General Assembly, Helsinki, Finland, June 1964, and amended by

The 29th WMA General Assembly, Tokyo, Japan, October 1975, 35th WMA General Assembly, Venice, Italy, October 1983, 41st WMA General Assembly, Hong Kong, September 1989, 48th WMA General Assembly, Somerset West, Republic of South Africa, October 1996, and the 52nd WMA General Assembly, Edinburgh, Scotland, October 2000, Note of Clarification on Paragraph 29 added by the WMA General Assembly, Washington 2002, Note of Clarification on Paragraph 30 added by the WMA General Assembly, Tokyo 2004

A. INTRODUCTION

1. The World Medical Association has developed the Declaration of Helsinki as a statement of ethical principles to provide guidance to physicians and other participants in medical research involving human subjects. Medical research involving human subjects includes research on identifiable human material or identifiable data.

2. It is the duty of the physician to promote and safeguard the health of the people. The physician's knowledge and conscience are dedicated to the fulfillment of this duty.

3. The Declaration of Geneva of the World Medical Association binds the physician with the words, "The health of my patient will be my first consideration," and the International Code of Medical Ethics declares that, "A physician shall act only in the patient's interest when providing medical care which might have the effect of weakening the physical and mental condition of the patient."

4. Medical progress is based on research which ultimately must rest in part on experimentation involving human subjects.

Clinical Trials Audit Preparation: A Guide for Good Clinical Practice (GCP) Inspections, by Vera Mihajlovic-Madzarevic
Copyright © 2010 John Wiley & Sons, Inc.

5. In medical research on human subjects, considerations related to the well-being of the human subject should take precedence over the interests of science and society.

6. The primary purpose of medical research involving human subjects is to improve prophylactic, diagnostic and therapeutic procedures and the understanding of the aetiology and pathogenesis of disease. Even the best proven prophylactic, diagnostic, and therapeutic methods must continuously be challenged through research for their effectiveness, efficiency, accessibility and quality.

7. In current medical practice and in medical research, most prophylactic, diagnostic and therapeutic procedures involve risks and burdens.

8. Medical research is subject to ethical standards that promote respect for all human beings and protect their health and rights. Some research populations are vulnerable and need special protection. The particular needs of the economically and medically disadvantaged must be recognized. Special attention is also required for those who cannot give or refuse consent for themselves, for those who may be subject to giving consent under duress, for those who will not benefit personally from the research and for those for whom the research is combined with care.

9. Research Investigators should be aware of the ethical, legal and regulatory requirements for research on human subjects in their own countries as well as applicable international requirements. No national ethical, legal or regulatory requirement should be allowed to reduce or eliminate any of the protections for human subjects set forth in this Declaration.

B. BASIC PRINCIPLES FOR ALL MEDICAL RESEARCH

10. It is the duty of the physician in medical research to protect the life, health, privacy, and dignity of the human subject.

11. Medical research involving human subjects must conform to generally accepted scientific principles, be based on a thorough knowledge of the scientific literature, other relevant sources of information, and on adequate laboratory and, where appropriate, animal experimentation.

12. Appropriate caution must be exercised in the conduct of research which may affect the environment, and the welfare of animals used for research must be respected.

13. The design and performance of each experimental procedure involving human subjects should be clearly formulated in an experimental protocol. This protocol should be submitted for consideration, comment, guidance, and where appropriate, approval to a specially appointed ethical review committee, which must be independent of the investigator, the sponsor or any other kind of undue influence. This independent committee should be in conformity with the laws and regulations of the country in which the research experiment is performed. The committee has the right to monitor ongoing trials. The researcher has the obligation to provide monitoring information to the committee, especially any serious adverse events. The researcher should also submit to the committee, for review, information regarding funding, sponsors, institutional affiliations, other potential conflicts of interest and incentives for subjects.

14. The research protocol should always contain a statement of the ethical considerations involved and should indicate that there is compliance with the principles enunciated in this Declaration.

15. Medical research involving human subjects should be conducted only by scientifically qualified persons and under the supervision of a clinically competent medical person. The responsibility for the human subject must always rest with a medically qualified person and never rest on the subject of the research, even though the subject has given consent.

16. Every medical research project involving human subjects should be preceded by careful assessment of predictable risks and burdens in comparison with foreseeable benefits to the subject or to others. This does not preclude the participation of healthy volunteers in medical research. The design of all studies should be publicly available.

17. Physicians should abstain from engaging in research projects involving human subjects unless they are confident that the risks involved have been adequately assessed and can be satisfactorily managed. Physicians should cease any investigation if the risks are found to outweigh the potential benefits or if there is conclusive proof of positive and beneficial results.

18. Medical research involving human subjects should only be conducted if the importance of the objective outweighs the inherent risks and burdens to the subject. This is especially important when the human subjects are healthy volunteers.

19. Medical research is only justified if there is a reasonable likelihood that the populations in which the research is carried out stand to benefit from the results of the research.

20. The subjects must be volunteers and informed participants in the research project.

21. The right of research subjects to safeguard their integrity must always be respected. Every precaution should be taken to respect the privacy of the subject, the confidentiality of the patient's information and to minimize the impact of the study on the subject's physical and mental integrity and on the personality of the subject.

22. In any research on human beings, each potential subject must be adequately informed of the aims, methods, sources of funding, any possible conflicts of interest, institutional affiliations of the researcher, the anticipated benefits and potential risks of the study and the discomfort it may entail. The subject should be informed of the right to abstain from participation in the study or to withdraw consent to participate at any time without reprisal. After ensuring that the subject has understood the information, the physician should then obtain the subject's freely-given informed consent, preferably in writing. If the consent cannot be obtained in writing, the non-written consent must be formally documented and witnessed.

23. When obtaining informed consent for the research project the physician should be particularly cautious if the subject is in a dependent relationship with the physician or may consent under duress. In that case the informed consent should be obtained by a well-informed physician who is not engaged in the investigation and who is completely independent of this relationship.

24. For a research subject who is legally incompetent, physically or mentally incapable of giving consent or is a legally incompetent minor, the investigator must obtain informed consent from the legally authorized representative in accordance with applicable law. These groups should not be included in research unless the research is necessary to promote the health of the population represented and this research cannot instead be performed on legally competent persons.

25. When a subject deemed legally incompetent, such as a minor child, is able to give assent to decisions about participation in research, the investigator must obtain that assent in addition to the consent of the legally authorized representative.

26. Research on individuals from whom it is not possible to obtain consent, including proxy or advance consent, should be done only if the physical/mental condition that prevents obtaining informed consent is a necessary characteristic of the research population. The specific reasons for involving research subjects with a condition that renders them unable to give informed consent should be stated in the experimental protocol for consideration and approval of the review committee. The protocol should state that consent to remain in the research should be obtained as soon as possible from the individual or a legally authorized surrogate.

27. Both authors and publishers have ethical obligations. In publication of the results of research, the investigators are obliged to preserve the accuracy of the results. Negative as well as positive results should be published or otherwise publicly available. Sources of funding, institutional affiliations and any possible conflicts of interest should be declared in the publication. Reports of experimentation not in accordance with the principles laid down in this Declaration should not be accepted for publication.

C. ADDITIONAL PRINCIPLES FOR MEDICAL RESEARCH COMBINED WITH MEDICAL CARE

28. The physician may combine medical research with medical care, only to the extent that the research is justified by its potential prophylactic, diagnostic or therapeutic value. When medical research is combined with medical care, additional standards apply to protect the patients who are research subjects.

29. The benefits, risks, burdens and effectiveness of a new method should be tested against those of the best current prophylactic, diagnostic, and therapeutic methods. This does not exclude the use of placebo, or no treatment, in studies where no proven prophylactic, diagnostic or therapeutic method exists.[1]

30. At the conclusion of the study, every patient entered into the study should be assured of access to the best proven prophylactic, diagnostic and therapeutic methods identified by the study.[2]

31. The physician should fully inform the patient which aspects of the care are related to the research. The refusal of a patient to participate in a study must never interfere with the patient-physician relationship.

32. In the treatment of a patient, where proven prophylactic, diagnostic and therapeutic methods do not exist or have been ineffective, the physician, with informed consent from the patient, must be free to use unproven or new prophylactic, diagnostic and therapeutic measures, if in the physician's judgment it offers hope of saving life, re-establishing health or alleviating suffering. Where possible, these measures should be made the object of research, designed to evaluate their safety and efficacy. In all cases, new information should be recorded and, where appropriate, published. The other relevant guidelines of this Declaration should be followed.

The WMA hereby reaffirms its position that extreme care must be taken in making use of a placebo-controlled trial and that in general this methodology should only be

[1] Note of clarification on paragraph 29 of the WMA Declaration of Helsinki
[2] Note of clarification on paragraph 30 of the WMA Declaration of Helsinki

used in the absence of existing proven therapy. However, a placebo-controlled trial may be ethically acceptable, even if proven therapy is available, under the following circumstances:

– Where for compelling and scientifically sound methodological reasons its use is necessary to determine the efficacy or safety of a prophylactic, diagnostic or therapeutic method; or

– Where a prophylactic, diagnostic or therapeutic method is being investigated for a minor condition and the patients who receive placebo will not be subject to any additional risk of serious or irreversible harm.

All other provisions of the Declaration of Helsinki must be adhered to, especially the need for appropriate ethical and scientific review.

The WMA hereby reaffirms its position that it is necessary during the study planning process to identify post-trial access by study participants to prophylactic, diagnostic and therapeutic procedures identified as beneficial in the study or access to other appropriate care. Post-trial access arrangements or other care must be described in the study protocol so the ethical review committee may consider such arrangements during its review.

9.10.2004

NUREMBERG CODE*

1. The voluntary consent of the human subject is absolutely essential. This means that the person involved should have legal capacity to give consent; should be so situated as to be able to exercise free power of choice, without the intervention of any element of force, fraud, deceit, duress, over-reaching, or other ulterior form of constraint or coercion; and should have sufficient knowledge and comprehension of the elements of the subject matter involved as to enable him to make an understanding and enlightened decision. This latter element requires that before the acceptance of an affirmative decision by the experimental subject there should be made known to him the nature, duration, and purpose of the experiment; the method and means by which it is to be conducted; all inconveniences and hazards reasonable to be expected; and the effects upon his health or person which may possibly come from his participation in the experiment.

   The duty and responsibility for ascertaining the quality of the consent rests upon each individual who initiates, directs or engages in the experiment. It is a personal duty and responsibility which may not be delegated to another with impunity.

2. The experiment should be such as to yield fruitful results for the good of society, unprocurable by other methods or means of study, and not random and unnecessary in nature.

3. The experiment should be so designed and based on the results of animal experimentation and a knowledge of the natural history of the disease or other problem under study that the anticipated results will justify the performance of the experiment.

4. The experiment should be so conducted as to avoid all unnecessary physical and mental suffering and injury.

5. No experiment should be conducted where there is an a priori reason to believe that death or disabling injury will occur; except, perhaps, in those experiments where the experimental physicians also serve as subjects.

6. The degree of risk to be taken should never exceed that determined by the humanitarian importance of the problem to be solved by the experiment.

---

*Reprinted from *Trials of War Criminals before the Nuremberg Military Tribunals under Control Council Law No. 10*, **Vol. 2, pp. 181–182**. Washington, DC: U.S. Government Printing Office, 1949.

---

7. Proper preparations should be made and adequate facilities provided to protect the experimental subject against even remote possibilities of injury, disability, or death.

8. The experiment should be conducted only by scientifically qualified persons. The highest degree of skill and care should be required through all stages of the experiment of those who conduct or engage in the experiment.

9. During the course of the experiment the human subject should be at liberty to bring the experiment to an end if he has reached the physical or mental state where continuation of the experiment seems to him to be impossible.

10. During the course of the experiment the scientist in charge must be prepared to terminate the experiment at any stage, if he has probable cause to believe, in the exercise of the good faith, superior skill and careful judgment required of him that a continuation of the experiment is likely to result in injury, disability, or death to the experimental subject.

THE BELMONT REPORT: ETHICAL PRINCIPLES AND GUIDELINES FOR THE PROTECTION OF HUMAN SUBJECTS OF RESEARCH

The National Commission for the Protection of Human Subjects of Biomedical and Behavioral Research April 18, 1979

AGENCY: Department of Health, Education, and Welfare.

ACTION: Notice of Report for Public Comment.

SUMMARY: On July 12, 1974, the National Research Act (Pub. L. 93-348) was signed into law, there-by creating the National Commission for the Protection of Human Subjects of Biomedical and Behavioral Research. One of the charges to the Commission was to identify the basic ethical principles that should underlie the conduct of biomedical and behavioral research involving human subjects and to develop guidelines which should be followed to assure that such research is conducted in accordance with those principles. In carrying out the above, the Commission was directed to consider: **(i)** the boundaries between biomedical and behavioral research and the accepted and routine practice of medicine, **(ii)** the role of assessment of risk-benefit criteria in the determination of the appropriateness of research involving human subjects, **(iii)** appropriate guidelines for the selection of human subjects for participation in such research and **(iv)** the nature and definition of informed consent in various research settings.

The Belmont Report attempts to summarize the basic ethical principles identified by the Commission in the course of its deliberations. It is the outgrowth of an intensive four-day period of discussions that were held in February 1976 at the Smithsonian Institution's Belmont Conference Center supplemented by the monthly deliberations of the Commission that were held over a period of nearly four years. It is a statement of basic ethical principles and guidelines that should assist in resolving the ethical problems that surround the conduct of research with human subjects. By publishing the Report in the Federal Register, and providing reprints upon request, the Secretary intends that it may be made readily available to scientists, members of Institutional Review Boards, and Federal employees. The two-volume Appendix, containing the lengthy reports of experts and specialists who assisted the Commission in fulfilling this part of its charge,

Clinical Trials Audit Preparation: A Guide for Good Clinical Practice (GCP) Inspections, by Vera Mihajlovic-Madzarevic
Copyright © 2010 John Wiley & Sons, Inc.

is available as DHEW Publication No. (OS) 78-0013 and No. (OS) 78-0014, for sale by the Superintendent of Documents, U.S. Government Printing Office, Washington, D.C. 20402.

Unlike most other reports of the Commission, the Belmont Report does not make specific recommendations for administrative action by the Secretary of Health, Education, and Welfare. Rather, the Commission recommended that the Belmont Report be adopted in its entirety, as a statement of the Department's policy. The Department requests public comment on this recommendation.

National Commission for the Protection of Human Subjects of
Biomedical and Behavioral Research

Members of the Commission

Kenneth John Ryan, M.D., Chairman, Chief of Staff, Boston Hospital for Women.
Joseph V. Brady, Ph.D., Professor of Behavioral Biology, Johns Hopkins University.
Robert E. Cooke, M.D., President, Medical College of Pennsylvania.
Dorothy I. Height, President, National Council of Negro Women, Inc.
Albert R. Jonsen, Ph.D., Associate Professor of Bioethics, University of California at San Francisco.
Patricia King, J.D., Associate Professor of Law, Georgetown University Law Center.
Karen Lebacqz, Ph.D., Associate Professor of Christian Ethics, Pacific School of Religion.
*** David W. Louisell, J.D., Professor of Law, University of California at Berkeley.
Donald W. Seldin, M.D., Professor and Chairman, Department of Internal Medicine, University of Texas at Dallas.
Eliot Stellar, Ph.D., Provost of the University and Professor of Physiological Psychology, University of Pennsylvania.
*** Robert H. Turtle, LL.B., Attorney, VomBaur, Coburn, Simmons & Turtle, Washington, D.C.
*** Deceased.

Table of Contents
Ethical Principles and Guidelines for Research Involving Human Subjects

A. *Boundaries Between Practice and Research*

B. *Basic Ethical Principles*

   2.1 *Respect for Persons*

   2.2 *Beneficence*

   2.3 *Justice*

C. *Applications*

   3.1 *Informed Consent*

   3.2 *Assessment of Risk and Benefits*

   3.3 *Selection of Subjects*

Ethical Principles and Guidelines for Research Involving Human Subjects
Scientific research has produced substantial social benefits. It has also posed some troubling ethical questions. Public attention was drawn to these questions by reported

abuses of human subjects in biomedical experiments, especially during the Second World War. During the Nuremberg War Crime Trials, the Nuremberg code was drafted as a set of standards for judging physicians and scientists who had conducted biomedical experiments on concentration camp prisoners. This code became the prototype of many later codes [1] intended to assure that research involving human subjects would be carried out in an ethical manner.

The codes consist of rules, some general, others specific, that guide the investigators or the reviewers of research in their work. Such rules often are inadequate to cover complex situations; at times they come into conflict, and they are frequently difficult to interpret or apply. Broader ethical principles will provide a basis on which specific rules may be formulated, criticized and interpreted.

Three principles, or general prescriptive judgments, that are relevant to research involving human subjects are identified in this statement. Other principles may also be relevant. These three are comprehensive, however, and are stated at a level of generalization that should assist scientists, subjects, reviewers and interested citizens to understand the ethical issues inherent in research involving human subjects. These principles cannot always be applied so as to resolve beyond dispute particular ethical problems. The objective is to provide an analytical framework that will guide the resolution of ethical problems arising from research involving human subjects.

This statement consists of a distinction between research and practice, a discussion of the three basic ethical principles, and remarks about the application of these principles.

PART A: BOUNDARIES BETWEEN PRACTICE AND RESEARCH

A. Boundaries Between Practice and Research

It is important to distinguish between biomedical and behavioral research, on the one hand, and the practice of accepted therapy on the other, in order to know what activities ought to undergo review for the protection of human subjects of research. The distinction between research and practice is blurred partly because both often occur together (as in research designed to evaluate a therapy) and partly because notable departures from standard practice are often called "experimental" when the terms "experimental" and "research" are not carefully defined.

For the most part, the term "practice" refers to interventions that are designed solely to enhance the well-being of an individual patient or client and that have a reasonable expectation of success. The purpose of medical or behavioral practice is to provide diagnosis, preventive treatment or therapy to particular individuals [2]. By contrast, the term "research' designates an activity designed to test an hypothesis, permit conclusions to be drawn, and thereby to develop or contribute to generalizable knowledge (expressed, for example, in theories, principles, and statements of relationships). Research is usually described in a formal protocol that sets forth an objective and a set of procedures designed to reach that objective.

When a clinician departs in a significant way from standard or accepted practice, the innovation does not, in and of itself, constitute research. The fact that a procedure is "experimental," in the sense of new, untested or different, does not automatically place it in the category of research. Radically new procedures of this description should, however, be made the object of formal research at an early stage in order to determine whether they are safe and effective. Thus, it is the responsibility of medical practice committees, for example, to insist that a major innovation be incorporated into a formal research project [3].

Research and practice may be carried on together when research is designed to evaluate the safety and efficacy of a therapy. This need not cause any confusion regarding whether or not the activity requires review; the general rule is that if there is any element of research in an activity, that activity should undergo review for the protection of human subjects.

PART B: BASIC ETHICAL PRINCIPLES

B. Basic Ethical Principles

The expression "basic ethical principles" refers to those general judgments that serve as a basic justification for the many particular ethical prescriptions and evaluations of human actions. Three basic principles, among those generally accepted in our cultural tradition, are particularly relevant to the ethics of research involving human subjects: the principles of respect of persons, beneficence and justice.

1. **Respect for Persons.**—Respect for persons incorporates at least two ethical convictions: first, that individuals should be treated as autonomous agents, and second, that persons with diminished autonomy are entitled to protection. The principle of respect for persons thus divides into two separate moral requirements: the requirement to acknowledge autonomy and the requirement to protect those with diminished autonomy.

An autonomous person is an individual capable of deliberation about personal goals and of acting under the direction of such deliberation. To respect autonomy is to give weight to autonomous persons' considered opinions and choices while refraining from obstructing their actions unless they are clearly detrimental to others. To show lack of respect for an autonomous agent is to repudiate that person's considered judgments, to deny an individual the freedom to act on those considered judgments, or to withhold information necessary to make a considered judgment, when there are no compelling reasons to do so.

However, not every human being is capable of self-determination. The capacity for self-determination matures during an individual's life, and some individuals lose this capacity wholly or in part because of illness, mental disability, or circumstances that severely restrict liberty. Respect for the immature and the incapacitated may require protecting them as they mature or while they are incapacitated.

Some persons are in need of extensive protection, even to the point of excluding them from activities which may harm them; other persons require little protection beyond making sure they undertake activities freely and with awareness of possible adverse consequence. The extent of protection afforded should depend upon the risk of harm and the likelihood of benefit. The judgment that any individual lacks autonomy should be periodically reevaluated and will vary in different situations.

In most cases of research involving human subjects, respect for persons demands that subjects enter into the research voluntarily and with adequate information. In some situations, however, application of the principle is not obvious. The involvement of prisoners as subjects of research provides an instructive example. On the one hand, it would seem that the principle of respect for persons requires that prisoners not be deprived of the opportunity to volunteer for research. On the other hand, under prison conditions they may be subtly coerced or unduly influenced to engage in research activities for which they would not otherwise volunteer. Respect for persons would then dictate that prisoners be protected. Whether to allow prisoners to "volunteer" or to "protect" them presents a dilemma. Respecting persons, in most hard cases, is often a matter of balancing competing claims urged by the principle of respect itself.

2. **Beneficence.**—Persons are treated in an ethical manner not only by respecting their decisions and protecting them from harm, but also by making efforts to secure their well-being. Such treatment falls under the principle of beneficence. The term "beneficence" is often understood to cover acts of kindness or charity that go beyond strict obligation. In this document, beneficence is understood in a stronger sense, as an obligation. Two general rules have been formulated as complementary expressions of beneficent actions in this sense: (1) do not harm and (2) maximize possible benefits and minimize possible harms.

The Hippocratic maxim "do no harm" has long been a fundamental principle of medical ethics. Claude Bernard extended it to the realm of research, saying that one should not injure one person regardless of the benefits that might come to others. However, even avoiding harm requires learning what is harmful; and, in the process of obtaining this information, persons may be exposed to risk of harm. Further, the Hippocratic Oath requires physicians to benefit their patients "according to their best judgment." Learning what will in fact benefit may require exposing persons to risk. The problem posed by these imperatives is to decide when it is justifiable to seek certain benefits despite the risks involved, and when the benefits should be foregone because of the risks.

The obligations of beneficence affect both individual investigators and society at large, because they extend both to particular research projects and to the entire enterprise of research. In the case of particular projects, investigators and members of their institutions are obliged to give forethought to the maximization of benefits and the reduction of risk that might occur from the research investigation. In the case of scientific research in general, members of the larger society are obliged to recognize the longer term benefits and risks that may result from the improvement of knowledge and from the development of novel medical, psychotherapeutic, and social procedures.

The principle of beneficence often occupies a well-defined justifying role in many areas of research involving human subjects. An example is found in research involving children. Effective ways of treating childhood diseases and fostering healthy development are benefits that serve to justify research involving children—even when individual research subjects are not direct beneficiaries. Research also makes it possible to avoid the harm that may result from the application of previously accepted routine practices that on closer investigation turn out to be dangerous. But the role of the principle of beneficence is not always so unambiguous. A difficult ethical problem remains, for example, about research that presents more than minimal risk without immediate prospect of direct benefit to the children involved. Some have argued that such research is inadmissible, while others have pointed out that this limit would rule out much research promising great benefit to children in the future. Here again, as with all hard cases, the different claims covered by the principle of beneficence may come into conflict and force difficult choices.

3. **Justice.**—Who ought to receive the benefits of research and bear its burdens? This is a question of justice, in the sense of "fairness in distribution" or "what is deserved."

An injustice occurs when some benefit to which a person is entitled is denied without good reason or when some burden is imposed unduly. Another way of conceiving the principle of justice is that equals ought to be treated equally. However, this statement requires explication. Who is equal and who is unequal? What considerations justify departure from equal distribution? Almost all commentators allow that distinctions based on experience, age, deprivation, competence, merit and position do sometimes constitute criteria justifying differential treatment for certain purposes. It is necessary, then, to explain in what respects people should be treated equally. There are several widely accepted formulations of just ways to distribute burdens and benefits. Each formulation mentions some relevant property on the basis of which burdens and benefits should be distributed. These formulations are (1) to each person an equal share, (2) to each person according to individual need, (3) to each person according to individual effort, (4) to each person according to societal contribution, and (5) to each person according to merit.

Questions of justice have long been associated with social practices such as punishment, taxation and political representation. Until recently these questions have not generally been associated with scientific research. However, they are foreshadowed even in the earliest reflections on the ethics of research involving human subjects. For example, during the 19th and early 20th centuries the burdens of serving as research subjects fell largely upon poor ward patients, while the benefits of improved medical care flowed primarily to private patients. Subsequently, the exploitation of unwilling prisoners as research subjects in Nazi concentration camps was condemned as a particularly flagrant injustice. In this country, in the 1940's, the Tuskegee syphilis study used disadvantaged, rural black men to study the untreated course of a disease that is by no means confined to that population. These subjects were deprived of demonstrably effective treatment in order not to interrupt the project, long after such treatment became generally available.

Against this historical background, it can be seen how conceptions of justice are relevant to research involving human subjects. For example, the selection of research subjects needs to be scrutinized in order to determine whether some classes (e.g., welfare patients, particular racial and ethnic minorities, or persons confined to institutions) are being systematically selected simply because of their easy availability, their compromised position, or their manipulability, rather than for reasons directly related to the problem being studied. Finally, whenever research supported by public funds leads to the development of therapeutic devices and procedures, justice demands both that these not provide advantages only to those who can afford them and that such research should not unduly involve persons from groups unlikely to be among the beneficiaries of subsequent applications of the research.

PART C: APPLICATIONS

C. Applications

Applications of the general principles to the conduct of research leads to consideration of the following requirements: informed consent, risk/benefit assessment, and the selection of subjects of research.

1. **Informed Consent.**—Respect for persons requires that subjects, to the degree that they are capable, be given the opportunity to choose what shall or shall not happen

to them. This opportunity is provided when adequate standards for informed consent are satisfied.

While the importance of informed consent is unquestioned, controversy prevails over the nature and possibility of an informed consent. Nonetheless, there is widespread agreement that the consent process can be analyzed as containing three elements: information, comprehension and voluntariness.

Information. Most codes of research establish specific items for disclosure intended to assure that subjects are given sufficient information. These items generally include: the research procedure, their purposes, risks and anticipated benefits, alternative procedures (where therapy is involved), and a statement offering the subject the opportunity to ask questions and to withdraw at any time from the research. Additional items have been proposed, including how subjects are selected, the person responsible for the research, etc.

However, a simple listing of items does not answer the question of what the standard should be for judging how much and what sort of information should be provided. One standard frequently invoked in medical practice, namely the information commonly provided by practitioners in the field or in the locale, is inadequate since research takes place precisely when a common understanding does not exist. Another standard, currently popular in malpractice law, requires the practitioner to reveal the information that reasonable persons would wish to know in order to make a decision regarding their care. This, too, seems insufficient since the research subject, being in essence a volunteer, may wish to know considerably more about risks gratuitously undertaken than do patients who deliver themselves into the hand of a clinician for needed care. It may be that a standard of "the reasonable volunteer" should be proposed: the extent and nature of information should be such that persons, knowing that the procedure is neither necessary for their care nor perhaps fully understood, can decide whether they wish to participate in the furthering of knowledge. Even when some direct benefit to them is anticipated, the subjects should understand clearly the range of risk and the voluntary nature of participation.

A special problem of consent arises where informing subjects of some pertinent aspect of the research is likely to impair the validity of the research. In many cases, it is sufficient to indicate to subjects that they are being invited to participate in research of which some features will not be revealed until the research is concluded. In all cases of research involving incomplete disclosure, such research is justified only if it is clear that (1) incomplete disclosure is truly necessary to accomplish the goals of the research, (2) there are no undisclosed risks to subjects that are more than minimal, and (3) there is an adequate plan for debriefing subjects, when appropriate, and for dissemination of research results to them. Information about risks should never be withheld for the purpose of eliciting the cooperation of subjects, and truthful answers should always be given to direct questions about the research. Care should be taken to distinguish cases in which disclosure would destroy or invalidate the research from cases in which disclosure would simply inconvenience the investigator.

Comprehension. The manner and context in which information is conveyed is as important as the information itself. For example, presenting information in a disorganized and rapid fashion, allowing too little time for consideration or curtailing opportunities for questioning, all may adversely affect a subject's ability to make an informed choice.

Because the subject's ability to understand is a function of intelligence, rationality, maturity and language, it is necessary to adapt the presentation of the information to the subject's capacities. Investigators are responsible for ascertaining that the subject has comprehended the information. While there is always an obligation to ascertain that the information about risk to subjects is complete and adequately comprehended, when the risks are more serious, that obligation increases. On occasion, it may be suitable to give some oral or written tests of comprehension.

Special provision may need to be made when comprehension is severely limited—for example, by conditions of immaturity or mental disability. Each class of subjects that one might consider as incompetent (e.g., infants and young children, mentally disabled patients, the terminally ill and the comatose) should be considered on its own terms. Even for these persons, however, respect requires giving them the opportunity to choose to the extent they are able, whether or not to participate in research. The objections of these subjects to involvement should be honored, unless the research entails providing them a therapy unavailable elsewhere. Respect for persons also requires seeking the permission of other parties in order to protect the subjects from harm. Such persons are thus respected both by acknowledging their own wishes and by the use of third parties to protect them from harm.

The third parties chosen should be those who are most likely to understand the incompetent subject's situation and to act in that person's best interest. The person authorized to act on behalf of the subject should be given an opportunity to observe the research as it proceeds in order to be able to withdraw the subject from the research, if such action appears in the subject's best interest.

Voluntariness. An agreement to participate in research constitutes a valid consent only if voluntarily given. This element of informed consent requires conditions free of coercion and undue influence. Coercion occurs when an overt threat of harm is intentionally presented by one person to another in order to obtain compliance. Undue influence, by contrast, occurs through an offer of an excessive, unwarranted, inappropriate or improper reward or other overture in order to obtain compliance. Also, inducements that would ordinarily be acceptable may become undue influences if the subject is especially vulnerable.

Unjustifiable pressures usually occur when persons in positions of authority or commanding influence—especially where possible sanctions are involved—urge a course of action for a subject. A continuum of such influencing factors exists, however, and it is impossible to state precisely where justifiable persuasion ends and undue influence begins. But undue influence would include actions such as manipulating a person's choice through the controlling influence of a close relative and threatening to withdraw health services to which an individual would otherwise be entitled.

2. **Assessment of Risks and Benefits.**—The assessment of risks and benefits requires a careful arrayal of relevant data, including, in some cases, alternative ways of obtaining the benefits sought in the research. Thus, the assessment presents both an opportunity and a responsibility to gather systematic and comprehensive information about proposed research. For the investigator, it is a means to examine whether the proposed research is properly designed. For a review committee, it is a method for determining whether the risks that will be presented to subjects are justified. For prospective subjects, the assessment will assist the determination whether or not to participate.

The Nature and Scope of Risks and Benefits. The requirement that research be justified on the basis of a favorable risk/benefit assessment bears a close relation to the principle of beneficence, just as the moral requirement that informed consent be obtained is derived primarily from the principle of respect for persons. The term "risk" refers to a possibility that harm may occur. However, when expressions such as "small risk" or "high risk" are used, they usually refer (often ambiguously) both to the chance (probability) of experiencing a harm and the severity (magnitude) of the envisioned harm.

The term "benefit" is used in the research context to refer to something of positive value related to health or welfare. Unlike "risk," "benefit" is not a term that expresses probabilities. Risk is properly contrasted to probability of benefits, and benefits are properly contrasted with harms rather than risks of harm. Accordingly, so-called risk/benefit assessments are concerned with the probabilities and magnitudes of possible harm and anticipated benefits. Many kinds of possible harms and benefits need to be taken into account. There are, for example, risks of psychological harm, physical harm, legal harm, social harm and economic harm and the corresponding benefits. While the most likely types of harms to research subjects are those of psychological or physical pain or injury, other possible kinds should not be overlooked.

Risks and benefits of research may affect the individual subjects, the families of the individual subjects, and society at large (or special groups of subjects in society). Previous codes and Federal regulations have required that risks to subjects be outweighed by the sum of both the anticipated benefit to the subject, if any, and the anticipated benefit to society in the form of knowledge to be gained from the research. In balancing these different elements, the risks and benefits affecting the immediate research subject will normally carry special weight. On the other hand, interests other than those of the subject may on some occasions be sufficient by themselves to justify the risks involved in the research, so long as the subjects' rights have been protected. Beneficence thus requires that we protect against risk of harm to subjects and also that we be concerned about the loss of the substantial benefits that might be gained from research.

The Systematic Assessment of Risks and Benefits. It is commonly said that benefits and risks must be "balanced" and shown to be "in a favorable ratio." The metaphorical character of these terms draws attention to the difficulty of making precise judgments. Only on rare occasions will quantitative techniques be available for the scrutiny of research protocols. However, the idea of systematic, nonarbitrary analysis of risks and benefits should be emulated insofar as possible. This ideal requires those making decisions about the justifiability of research to be thorough in the accumulation and assessment of information about all aspects of the research, and to consider alternatives systematically. This procedure renders the assessment of research more rigorous and precise, while making communication between review board members and investigators less subject to misinterpretation, misinformation and conflicting judgments. Thus, there should first be a determination of the validity of the presuppositions of the research; then the nature, probability and magnitude of risk should be distinguished with as much clarity as possible. The method of ascertaining risks should be explicit, especially where there is no alternative to the use of such vague categories as small or slight risk. It should also be determined whether an investigator's estimates of the probability of harm or benefits are reasonable, as judged by known facts or other available studies.

Finally, assessment of the justifiability of research should reflect at least the following considerations: **(i)** Brutal or inhumane treatment of human subjects is never morally justified. **(ii)** Risks should be reduced to those necessary to achieve the research objective. It should be determined whether it is in fact necessary to use human subjects at all. Risk can perhaps never be entirely eliminated, but it can often be reduced by careful attention to alternative procedures. **(iii)** When research involves significant risk of serious impairment, review committees should be extraordinarily insistent on the justification of the risk (looking usually to the likelihood of benefit to the subject—or, in some rare cases, to the manifest voluntariness of the participation). (iv) When vulnerable populations are involved in research, the appropriateness of involving them should itself be demonstrated. A number of variables go into such judgments, including the nature and degree of risk, the condition of the particular population involved, and the nature and level of the anticipated benefits. (v) Relevant risks and benefits must be thoroughly arrayed in documents and procedures used in the informed consent process.

3. **Selection of Subjects.**—Just as the principle of respect for persons finds expression in the requirements for consent, and the principle of beneficence in risk/benefit assessment, the principle of justice gives rise to moral requirements that there be fair procedures and outcomes in the selection of research subjects.

Justice is relevant to the selection of subjects of research at two levels: the social and the individual. Individual justice in the selection of subjects would require that researchers exhibit fairness: thus, they should not offer potentially beneficial research only to some patients who are in their favor or select only "undesirable" persons for risky research. Social justice requires that distinction be drawn between classes of subjects that ought, and ought not, to participate in any particular kind of research, based on the ability of members of that class to bear burdens and on the appropriateness of placing further burdens on already burdened persons. Thus, it can be considered a matter of social justice that there is an order of preference in the selection of classes of subjects (e.g., adults before children) and that some classes of potential subjects (e.g., the institutionalized mentally infirm or prisoners) may be involved as research subjects, if at all, only on certain conditions.

Injustice may appear in the selection of subjects, even if individual subjects are selected fairly by investigators and treated fairly in the course of research. Thus injustice arises from social, racial, sexual and cultural biases institutionalized in society. Thus, even if individual researchers are treating their research subjects fairly, and even if IRBs are taking care to assure that subjects are selected fairly within a particular institution, unjust social patterns may nevertheless appear in the overall distribution of the burdens and benefits of research. Although individual institutions or investigators may not be able to resolve a problem that is pervasive in their social setting, they can consider distributive justice in selecting research subjects.

Some populations, especially institutionalized ones, are already burdened in many ways by their infirmities and environments. When research is proposed that involves risks and does not include a therapeutic component, other less burdened classes of persons should be called upon first to accept these risks of research, except where the research is directly related to the specific conditions of the class involved. Also, even though public funds for research may often flow in the same directions as public funds for health care, it seems unfair that populations dependent on public health care constitute a pool of preferred research subjects if more advantaged populations are likely to be the recipients of the benefits.

One special instance of injustice results from the involvement of vulnerable subjects. Certain groups, such as racial minorities, the economically disadvantaged, the very sick, and the institutionalized may continually be sought as research subjects, owing to their ready availability in settings where research is conducted. Given their dependent status and their frequently compromised capacity for free consent, they should be protected against the danger of being involved in research solely for administrative convenience, or because they are easy to manipulate as a result of their illness or socioeconomic condition.

[1] Since 1945, various codes for the proper and responsible conduct of human experimentation in medical research have been adopted by different organizations. The best known of these codes are the Nuremberg Code of 1947, the Helsinki Declaration of 1964 (revised in 1975), and the 1971 Guidelines (codified into Federal Regulations in 1974) issued by the U.S. Department of Health, Education, and Welfare Codes for the conduct of social and behavioral research have also been adopted, the best known being that of the American Psychological Association, published in 1973.

[2] Although practice usually involves interventions designed solely to enhance the well-being of a particular individual, interventions are sometimes applied to one individual for the enhancement of the well-being of another (e.g., blood donation, skin grafts, organ transplants) or an intervention may have the dual purpose of enhancing the well-being of a particular individual, and, at the same time, providing some benefit to others (e.g., vaccination, which protects both the person who is vaccinated and society generally). The fact that some forms of practice have elements other than immediate benefit to the individual receiving an intervention, however, should not confuse the general distinction between research and practice. Even when a procedure applied in practice may benefit some other person, it remains an intervention designed to enhance the well-being of a particular individual or groups of individuals; thus, it is practice and need not be reviewed as research.

[3] Because the problems related to social experimentation may differ substantially from those of biomedical and behavioral research, the Commission specifically declines to make any policy determination regarding such research at this time. Rather, the Commission believes that the problem ought to be addressed by one of its successor bodies.

INDEX

Clinical Trials Audit Preparation: A Guide for Good Clinical Practice (GCP) Inspections, by Vera Mihajlovic-Madzarevic
Copyright © 2010 John Wiley & Sons, Inc.